S0-AKP-054

Wound Care

made Incredibly Visual!™

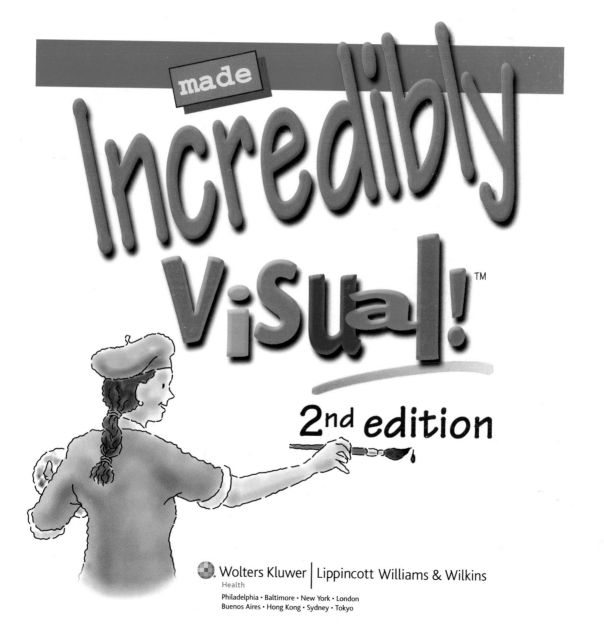

2nd edition

Wolters Kluwer | Lippincott Williams & Wilkins
Health

Philadelphia · Baltimore · New York · London
Buenos Aires · Hong Kong · Sydney · Tokyo

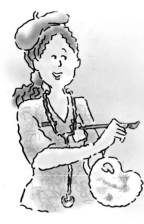

Staff

Publisher
J. Christopher Burghardt

Clinical Director
Joan M. Robinson, RN, MSN

Clinical Project Manager
Beverly Ann Tscheschlog, RN, MS

Clinical Editor
Joanne M. Bartelmo, RN, MSN

Product Director
David Moreau

Product Manager
Rosanne Hallowell

Editor
Jaime Stockslager Buss, MSPH, ELS

Copy Editors
Jerry Altobelli, Amy Furman

Editorial Assistants
Karen J. Kirk, Jeri O'Shea, Linda K. Ruhf

Art Director
Elaine Kasmer

Designer
Lynn Foulk

Design Assistant
Kate Zulak

Illustrators
Esteban Cabrera, Judy Newhouse,
Bot Roda, Betty Winnberg

Vendor Manager
Cindy Rudy

Manufacturing Manager
Beth J. Welsh

Production Services
SPi Global

The clinical treatments described and recommended in this publication are based on research and consultation with nursing, medical, and legal authorities. To the best of our knowledge, these procedures reflect currently accepted practice. Nevertheless, they can't be considered absolute and universal recommendations. For individual applications, all recommendations must be considered in light of the patient's clinical condition and, before administration of new or infrequently used drugs, in light of the latest package-insert information. The authors and publisher disclaim any responsibility for any adverse effects resulting from the suggested procedures, from any undetected errors, or from the reader's misunderstanding of the text.

© 2012 by Lippincott Williams & Wilkins. All rights reserved. This book is protected by copyright. No part of it may be reproduced, stored in a retrieval system, or transmitted, in any form or by any means—electronic, mechanical, photocopy, recording, or otherwise—without prior written permission of the publisher, except for brief quotations embodied in critical articles and reviews, and testing and evaluation materials provided by the publisher to instructors whose schools have adopted its accompanying textbook. For information, write Lippincott Williams & Wilkins, 323 Norristown Road, Suite 200, Ambler, PA 19002-2756.

Printed in China.

WCIV2E010511-020612

Library of Congress Cataloging-in-Publication Data

Wound care made incredibly visual. — Second Edition.
    p. ; cm.
    Includes bibliographical references and index.
    1. Wounds and injuries—Nursing—Handbooks, manuals, etc. 2. Wounds and injuries—Nursing—Atlases. I. Lippincott Williams & Wilkins, issuing body.
    [DNLM: 1. Wounds and Injuries—nursing—Atlases. 2. Wounds and Injuries—nursing—Handbooks. WY 49]
    RD93.95.W69 2011
    617.1—dc22
    ISBN 978-1-60913-620-8 (pbk.)   2010051104

Contents

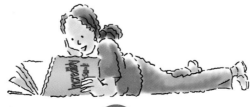

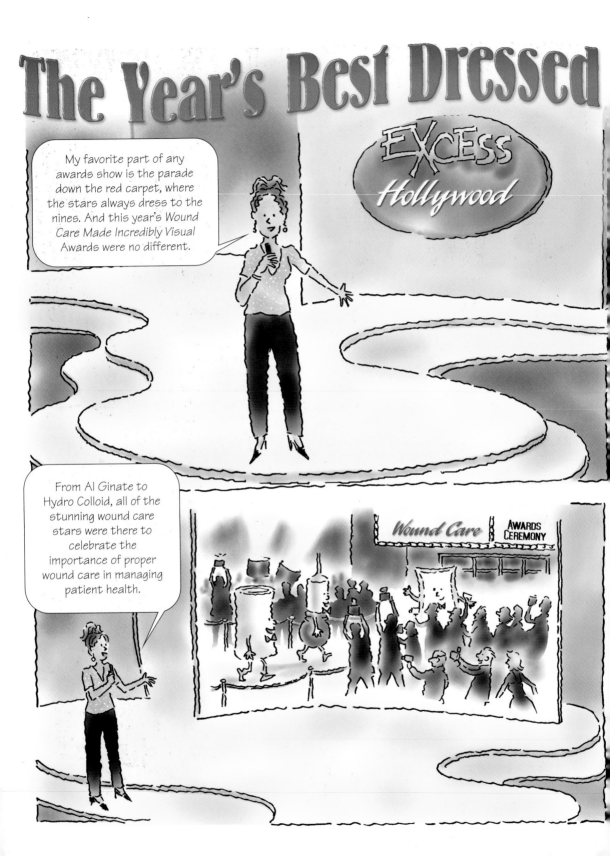

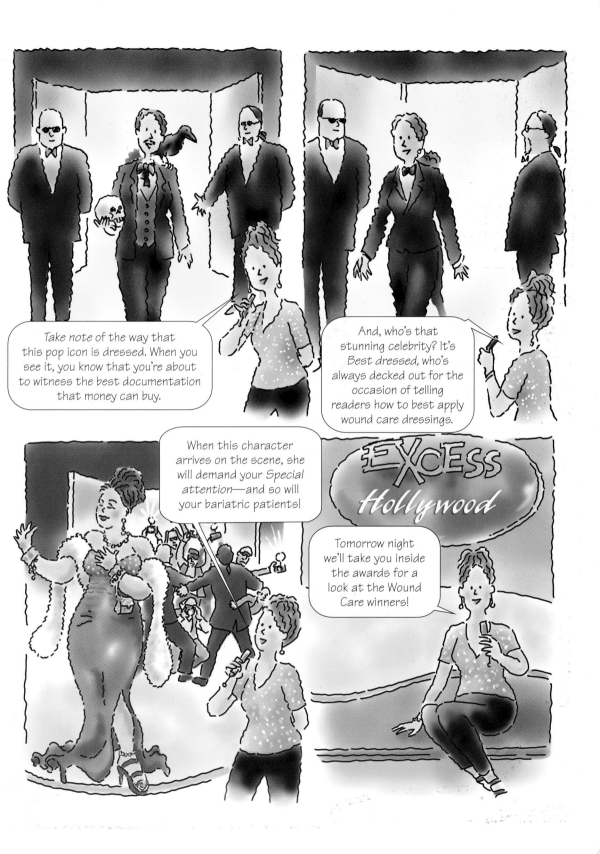

Contributors and consultants

Debbie Berry, RN, MSN, CPHQ, CWCN, CCCN
Vice President of Quality and Risk
Northside Hospital
St. Petersburg, Florida

Laura A. Conklin, RN, MSN, MSA, ONC, CWS, LNCC, FCCWS, DIP. AAWM
Professor
Wayne County Community College District
Detroit, Michigan

Evonne Fowler, RN, CWON
Certified Wound and Ostomy Nurse
San Gorgonio Hospital
Banning, California

Elizabeth R. Fudge, RN, MS, CWON
Wound/Ostomy RN
Wellstar Cobb Wound Care Center
Wellstar Cobb Hospital
Austell, Georgia

Julia Isen, RN, MS, FNP-C
Assistant Clinical Professor
UCSF Medical Center, Mt. Zion Campus
San Francisco, California

Jennifer L. Pettis, RN, WCC, RAC-MT
Consultant
Clifton Park, New York

Michelle C. Quigel, RN, BSN, CWOCN
Wound, Ostomy, Continence Nurse
Holy Redeemer Hospital and Medical Center
Meadowbrook, Pennsylvania

Tracy A. Robinson, RN, BSN, CWOCN
Home Health Nurse
MacNeal Home Care
Berwyn, Illinois

Tracey J. Siegel, MSN, RN, CWOCN, CNE
Instructor
Middlesex County Community College Nursing Program
Edison, New Jersey

Jennifer Smoltz, RN, MSN, CWOCN, ACNP-BC
Advanced Practice Nurse
University of Virginia Health System
Charlottesville, Virginia

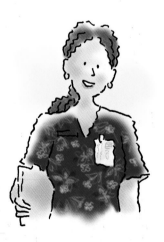

1
Skin anatomy and physiology

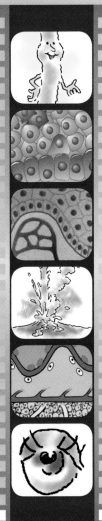

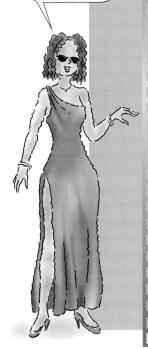

Beauty may be only skin deep, but in my line of work, that's important!

Anatomy

The skin, or integumentary system, is the largest organ in the body. It accounts for about 6 to 8 lb (2.5 to 3.5 kg) of a person's body weight and has a surface area of more than 20 square feet. The living cells in the skin receive oxygen and nutrients through an extensive network of small blood vessels.

Collaboration is key. Skin is made up of separate layers that function as a single unit.

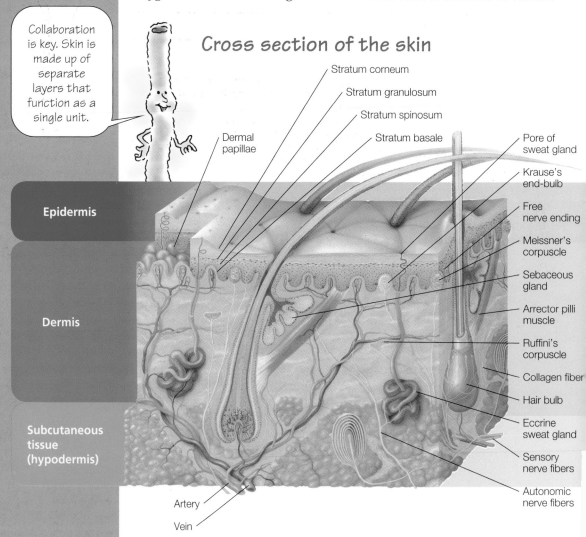

Cross section of the skin

- Stratum corneum
- Stratum granulosum
- Stratum spinosum
- Stratum basale
- Dermal papillae

- Pore of sweat gland
- Krause's end-bulb
- Free nerve ending
- Meissner's corpuscle
- Sebaceous gland
- Arrector pilli muscle
- Ruffini's corpuscle
- Collagen fiber
- Hair bulb
- Eccrine sweat gland
- Sensory nerve fibers
- Autonomic nerve fibers

- Artery
- Vein

Epidermis

Dermis

Subcutaneous tissue (hypodermis)

> Hair and sweat glands help stabilize the skin's structural networks.

Functions of the skin layers

Layer	Description
Epidermis	• Outermost layer • Consists of five sublayers • Formed mainly by keratinocytes (cells that are continuously generated and migrate from the underlying dermis and die upon reaching the surface) • Contains melanocytes (give skin and hair their color), Langerhans cells (provide the skin with immunological function), and Merkel cells (serve as markers of tactile function; confined to the lips and fingertips) • Regenerates itself every 4 to 6 weeks • Serves as a protective layer against water loss and physical damage
Dermis	• Composed of collagen fibers (give skin its strength), elastin fibers (provide elasticity), and an extracellular matrix (contributes to skin's strength and pliability) • Consists of two sublayers: the papillary dermis (outer layer composed of collagen and reticular fibers) and the reticular dermis (inner layer formed by thick networks of collagen bundles that anchor onto subcutaneous tissue and underlying support structures) • Contains blood and lymphatic vessels (supply nutrition and remove wastes), nerve fibers, hair follicles, sebaceous and sweat glands, and fibroblast cells (important in the production of collagen and elastin) • Supplies nutrition to the skin and supports the skin's structure and strength
Subcutaneous tissue (hypodermis)	• Subdermal layer of adipose and connective tissue • Contains major blood vessels, lymph vessels, and nerves • Insulates the body, absorbs shocks to the skeletal system, and helps skin move easily over underlying structures

A closer look at epidermal layers

The epidermis consists of five distinct layers. The innermost layer contains protrusions (called *rete pegs* or *epidermal ridges*) that extend down into the dermis. Surrounded by vascularized dermal papillae, these protrusions support the epidermis and facilitate the exchange of fluids and cells between skin layers.

> Let me get this straight: the skin has three main layers. Of those three layers, the outermost layer has five layers of its own. If that were a cake, I'd need a lot of icing.

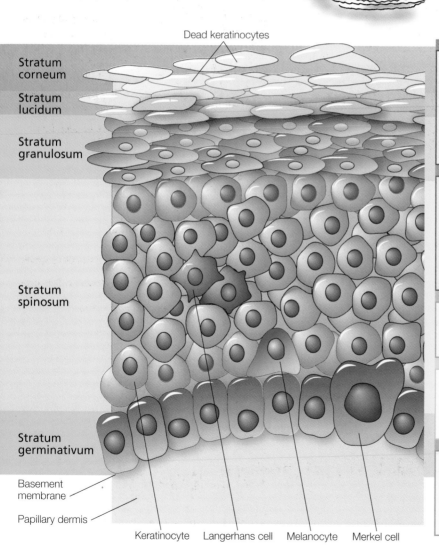

Dead keratinocytes

Stratum corneum

Stratum lucidum

Stratum granulosum

Stratum spinosum

Stratum germinativum

Basement membrane

Papillary dermis

Keratinocyte   Langerhans cell   Melanocyte   Merkel cell

The stratum corneum (a superficial layer of dead skin cells) has contact with the environment. The cells here shed daily and are replaced with cells from the layer beneath it.

The stratum lucidum (a single layer of cells) is most evident in areas where skin is thick—such as the palms and soles—and appears to be absent where skin is especially thin—such as the eyelids.

The stratum granulosum (one to five cells thick) aids keratin formation.

The stratum spinosum is where cells begin to flatten as they migrate toward the skin surface.

The stratum germinativum, or stratum basale, is one cell thick and is the only layer in which cells undergo mitosis to form new cells.

Blood supply

The skin receives its blood supply through vessels that originate in the underlying muscle. Here, arteries branch into smaller vessels, which then branch into the network of capillaries that permeate the dermis and subcutaneous tissue.

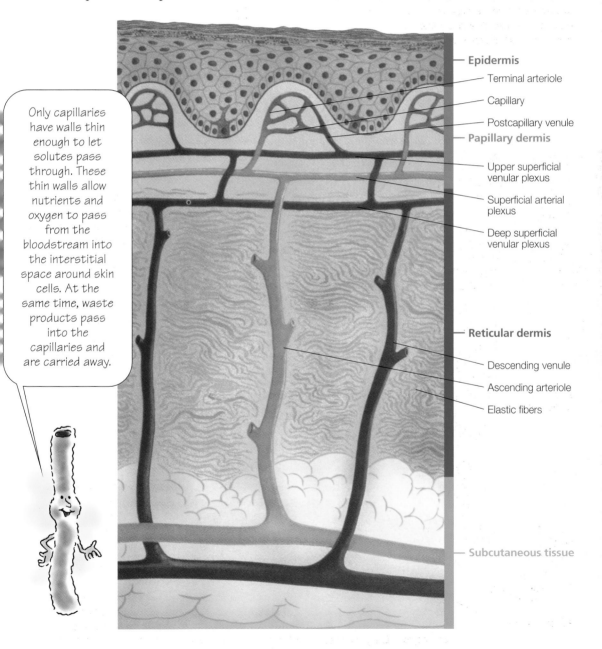

Only capillaries have walls thin enough to let solutes pass through. These thin walls allow nutrients and oxygen to pass from the bloodstream into the interstitial space around skin cells. At the same time, waste products pass into the capillaries and are carried away.

— **Epidermis**

Terminal arteriole

Capillary

Postcapillary venule

— **Papillary dermis**

Upper superficial venular plexus

Superficial arterial plexus

Deep superficial venular plexus

— **Reticular dermis**

Descending venule

Ascending arteriole

Elastic fibers

— **Subcutaneous tissue**

Physiology

Skin performs, or participates in, a host of vital functions. Damage to skin impairs its ability to carry out these important functions.

Functions of the skin

Function	Description
Protection	▪ Acts as a physical barrier to microorganisms and foreign matter, protecting the body against infection ▪ Protects underlying tissue and structures from mechanical injury ▪ Prevents the loss of water, electrolytes, proteins, and other substances
Sensory perception	▪ Contains nerve endings ▪ Allows for perception of pain, pressure, heat, and cold to identify potential dangers and avoid injury
Thermoregulation	▪ Contains nerves, blood vessels, and eccrine glands in the dermis to control body temperature ▪ Causes blood vessels to constrict (reducing blood flow and conserving heat) when exposed to cold or internal body temperature falls ▪ Causes small arteries in the skin to dilate and increases sweat production to promote cooling when skin becomes hot or internal body temperature rises
Excretion	▪ Transmits trace amounts of water and body wastes to the environment ▪ Allows the skin to maintain thermoregulation and electrolyte and hydration balances ▪ Prevents dehydration by ensuring that the body doesn't lose too much water
Metabolism	▪ Helps to maintain the mineralization of bones and teeth ▪ Synthesizes vitamin D (which is crucial to the metabolism of calcium and phosphate) when exposed to the ultraviolet spectrum in sunlight
Absorption	▪ Allows for the absorption of some drugs directly into the bloodstream

As people age, their skin's ability to sense pressure, heat, and cold becomes impaired, even though the number of nerve endings in the skin remains unchanged.

Aging and skin function

With aging, the skin undergoes a number of changes that increase the risk of wound development and impair the ability of wounds to heal.

Youthful skin

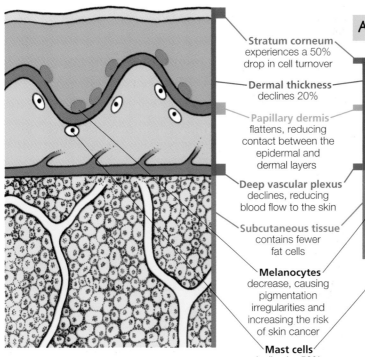

Aged skin

Stratum corneum experiences a 50% drop in cell turnover

Dermal thickness declines 20%

Papillary dermis flattens, reducing contact between the epidermal and dermal layers

Deep vascular plexus declines, reducing blood flow to the skin

Subcutaneous tissue contains fewer fat cells

Melanocytes decrease, causing pigmentation irregularities and increasing the risk of skin cancer

Mast cells decline by 50%, reducing the inflammatory response

VISION QUEST

Able to label?

Identify the five layers of the epidermis indicated on this illustration.

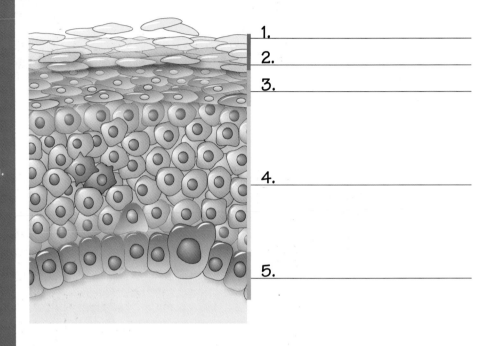

1. _____
2. _____
3. _____

4. _____

5. _____

Rebus riddle

Sound out each group of pictures and symbols to reveal an important fact about the skin.

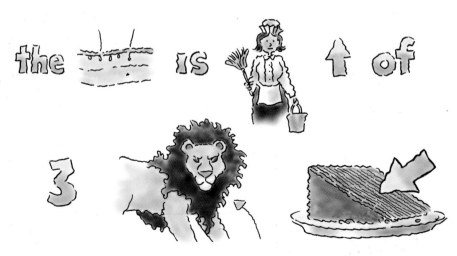

the [skin] is [maid] [↑] of

3 [lion] [cake↘]

Answers: Able to label? 1. Stratum corneum, 2. Stratum lucidum, 3. Stratum granulosum, 4. Stratum spinosum, 5. Stratum germinativum; Rebus riddle The skin is made up of three main layers.

2
Wound healing

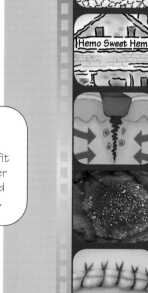

Trust me... sometimes things don't fit back together just like you'd like them to.

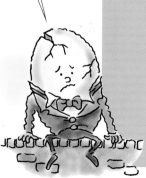

Types of wound healing

Any break in the skin is considered a wound. The extent and type of damage—as well as other intrinsic factors, such as patient circulation, nutrition, and hydration—influence the rate of wound repair. Wounds can heal, or close, through primary intention, secondary intention, or tertiary intention.

Primary intention

Wounds that heal through primary intention usually don't involve the loss of tissue. Examples include surgical wounds, superficial traumatic wounds, and first-degree sunburn.

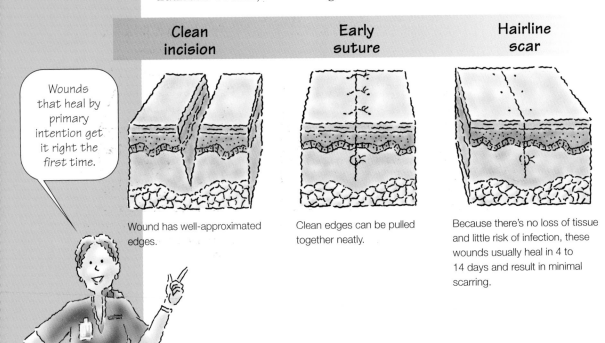

> Wounds that heal by primary intention get it right the first time.

Clean incision

Wound has well-approximated edges.

Early suture

Clean edges can be pulled together neatly.

Hairline scar

Because there's no loss of tissue and little risk of infection, these wounds usually heal in 4 to 14 days and result in minimal scarring.

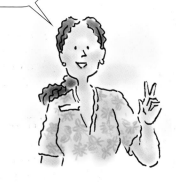

Wounds that heal by secondary intention need a second chance to get it right. Luckily, granulation tissue can "fill in" the gap.

Secondary intention

A wound that involves some degree of tissue loss heals by secondary intention. Pressure ulcers, burns, dehisced surgical wounds, and traumatic injuries are examples of this type of wound. These wounds take longer to heal, result in scarring, and have a higher rate of complications than wounds that heal by primary intention.

Gaping irregular wound	Granulation	Epithelium growth over scar
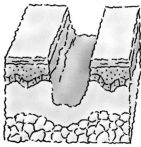	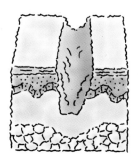	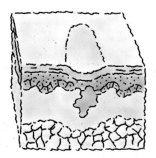
Edges can't be easily approximated.	Wound fills with granulation tissue.	A scar forms and reepithelialization occurs, primarily from the wound edges.

Tertiary intention

Wounds are sometimes left open for several days to allow edema or infection to resolve or for exudate to drain. These wounds heal by tertiary intention, also known as *delayed primary closure.* After the problem resolves, these wounds are closed with sutures or some other type of skin closure.

Open wound	Increased granulation	Late suturing with wide scar

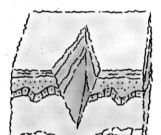 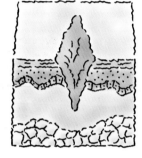 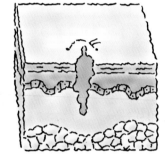

Wound is intentionally kept open (typically for 3 to 5 days) to allow edema or infection to resolve or to permit removal of exudate.

Wound fills with granulation tissue.

Wound is sutured late and a wide scar results.

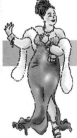

Special attention

Wound healing and bariatric patients

Bariatric patients are at risk for delayed wound healing due to:

■ reduced tissue perfusion in adipose tissue and increased tension at the suture line caused by the weight of excess body fat
■ excess skinfolds (especially if the wound is within a fold or if a fold covers a suture line, which may keep the wound moist and allow bacteria to accumulate)
■ associated medical conditions such as type 2 diabetes mellitus.

Bariatric patients are also at risk for dehiscence and evisceration because their diets may be seriously lacking in essential vitamins and minerals that are necessary for proper wound healing.

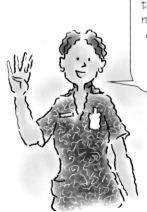

Wounds that heal by tertiary intention need three steps: draining, "filling" by granulation, and then suturing.

Phases of wound healing

The healing process is the same for all wounds, whether the cause is mechanical, chemical, or thermal. Health care professionals discuss the process of wound healing in four specific phases: hemostasis, inflammation, proliferation, and maturation.

Wound healing process

Injury

Hemostasis
Coagulation
Platelet aggregation
Beginning of growth factor secretion

Platelets

Inflammation
Macrophages
Neutrophils
Granulocytes

Neovascular growth
Acceleration of growth factor secretion

Wound cleansing
Debridement
Resistance to infection

Proliferation

Collagen lysis

Collagen synthesis

Granulation
Reepithelialization

Proteoglycan synthesis

Maturation
Remodeling

Contraction

Healed wound

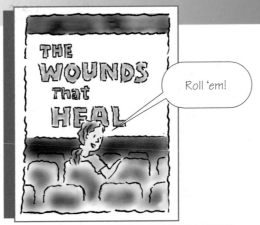

Hemostasis

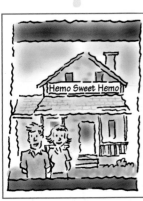

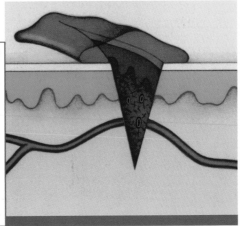

When tissue is damaged, serotonin, histamine, prostaglandins, and blood from the injured vessels fill the area. Blood platelets form a clot, and fibrin in the clot binds the wound edges together.

Inflammation

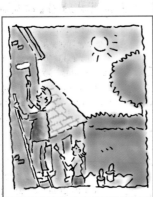

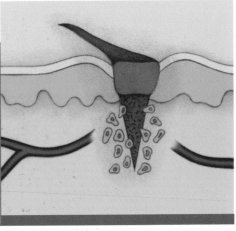

Lymphocytes initiate the inflammatory response, increasing capillary permeability. Wound edges swell. White blood cells from surrounding vessels move in and ingest bacteria and cellular debris, demolishing the clot and healing the wound. Redness, warmth, swelling, pain, and loss of function may occur. Platelets heavily secrete growth factors during this phase.

3 Proliferation

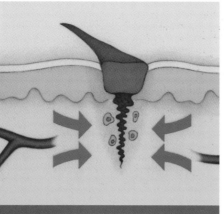

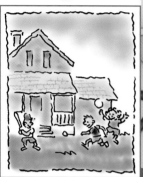

Adjacent healthy tissue supplies blood, nutrients, fibroblasts, proteins, and other building materials needed to form soft, pink, and highly vascular granulation tissue, which begins to fill and cover the area.

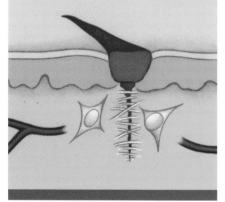

4 Maturation

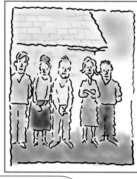

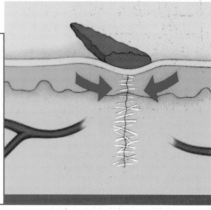

Fibroblasts in the granulation tissue secrete collagen, a gluelike substance. Collagen fibers crisscross the area, forming scar tissue. Meanwhile, epithelial cells at the wound edge multiply and migrate toward the wound center. A new layer of surface cells replaces the layer that was destroyed. New, healthy tissue or granulation tissue (if the blood supply is inadequate) appears.

Just as movies don't always reflect real life, healing rarely occurs in this strict order. Typically, the phases of wound healing overlap.

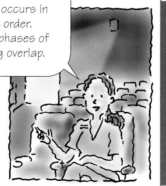

Over months or years, damaged tissue (including lymphatics, blood vessels, and stromal matrices) regenerates. Collagen fibers shorten, and the scar may diminish in size. Normal function may return, but the scar will only have approximately 80% of the strength of unwounded skin. Alternatively, the scar may hypertrophy, leading to the formation of a keloid and the development of contractures.

Recognizing wound failure to heal

Sign	Causes	Interventions
Wound bed		
Too dry	▪ Exposure of tissue and cells normally in a moist environment to air ▪ Inadequate hydration	▪ Add moisture regularly. ▪ Use a dressing that maintains moisture, such as a hydrocolloid or hydrogel dressing. ▪ Reassess patient hydration status.
No change in size or depth for 2 weeks	▪ Pressure or trauma to the area ▪ Poor nutrition, poor circulation, or inadequate hydration ▪ Poor control of disease processes such as diabetes ▪ Inadequate pain control ▪ Infection	▪ Reassess the patient for local or systemic problems that impair wound healing, and intervene as necessary.
Increase in size or depth	▪ Debridement ▪ Ischemia due to excess pressure or poor circulation ▪ Infection	▪ Reassess the patient for local or systemic problems that impair wound healing, and intervene as necessary. ▪ If caused by debridement, no intervention is necessary. ▪ Poor circulation may not be resolvable, but consider adding warmth to the area and administering a vasodilator or antiplatelet medication. ▪ If caused by infection, administer topical or systemic antimicrobials, as ordered.
Necrosis	▪ Ischemia	▪ Consult the medical provider regarding debridement if the remaining living tissue has adequate circulation.
Increase in drainage or change in drainage from clear to purulent	▪ Autolytic or enzymatic debridement ▪ Infection	▪ If caused by autolytic or enzymatic debridement, no intervention is necessary; an increase or change of color in drainage is expected because of the breakdown of dead tissue. ▪ If debridement isn't the cause, assess the wound for infection. ▪ If caused by infection, administer topical or systemic antimicrobials, as ordered.
Tunneling	▪ Pressure over bony prominences ▪ Presence of foreign body ▪ Deep infection	▪ Protect the area from pressure. ▪ Irrigate and inspect the tunnel as carefully as possible for a hidden suture or leftover bit of dressing material. ▪ If the tunnel doesn't shorten in length each week, thoroughly clean and obtain a tissue biopsy for infection and, with a chronic wound, for possible malignancy. ▪ Address potential causes of shear if the wound is a pressure ulcer.

Sometimes, no matter what you do, a plot just fails to come together.

Sign	Causes	Interventions
Wound edges		
Red, hot skin; tenderness; and induration	▪ Inflammation due to excess pressure or infection	▪ Protect the area from pressure. ▪ If pressure relief doesn't resolve the inflammation within 24 hours, topical antimicrobial therapy may be indicated.
Maceration (white skin)	▪ Excess moisture	▪ Protect the skin with petrolatum ointment or a barrier wipe. ▪ If practical, obtain an order for a more absorptive dressing.
Rolled skin edges	▪ Too-dry wound bed	▪ Obtain an order for moisture-retentive dressings. ▪ If rolling isn't resolved in 1 week, debridement of the edges may be necessary.
Undermining or ecchymosis of surrounding skin (loose or bruised skin edges)	▪ Excess shearing force to the area	▪ Protect the area from shear, especially during patient transfers. ▪ Address potential causes of shear.

Effects of aging on wound healing

Skin changes that occur with aging cause healing time to be prolonged in elderly patients.

Factors that delay healing

■ Slower turnover rate in epidermal cells
■ Poor oxygenation of the wound (due to increasingly fragile capillaries and a reduction in skin vascularization)
■ Impaired function of the respiratory or immune system
■ Reduced dermal and subcutaneous mass (leading to an increased risk of chronic pressure ulcers)
■ Lack of tensile strength in healed wounds, making them prone to reinjury

Factors that complicate healing

■ Poor nutrition and hydration
■ Presence of a chronic condition
■ Use of multiple medications, including antiinflammatory drugs
■ Decreased mobility
■ Incontinence

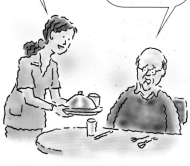

Physical changes from aging—such as a declining sense of smell and taste and decreased stomach motility—can affect a patient's nutritional and fluid intake.

Other factors can also affect our nutritional status, such as loose dentures, financial concerns, problems preparing or obtaining food, and mental status changes.

Complications of wound healing

Dehiscence and evisceration may require emergency surgery, especially when an abdominal wound is involved. If a wound opens without evisceration, it may need to heal by secondary intention.

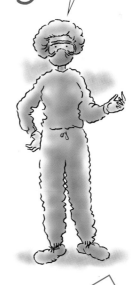

Wound dehiscence

Dehiscence is a separation of skin and tissue layers. It's most likely to occur 3 to 11 days after the injury was sustained and may follow surgery.

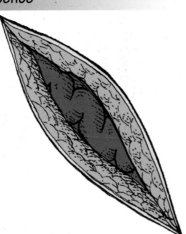

Evisceration of bowel loop

Evisceration is similar to dehiscence but involves protrusion of underlying visceral organs as well.

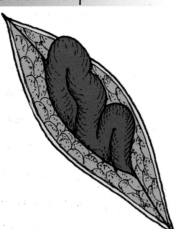

Poor nutrition and advanced age increase a patient's risk of dehiscence and evisceration.

Detecting wound dehiscence

Signs of dehiscence include an abscess or a gush of serosanguineous fluid from the wound. The patient may also report a "popping" sensation at the wound site.

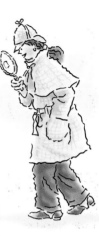

Dehisced abdominal wound (with a colostomy)

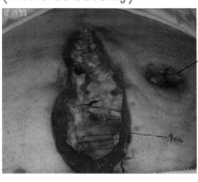

Dehisced healing abdominal incision

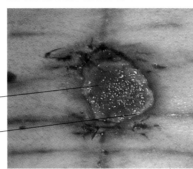

Colostomy

Red granulation tissue

Yellow fibrin slough

take note

Documenting wound dehiscence and evisceration

5/24/11	0945	During dressing change at 0925, noted dehiscence of distal 2" of midline abdominal incision. Superficial layers of tissue observed; no evisceration noted. Pt. placed in reclined position with knees flexed. Pt. states, "I felt something give when I coughed." Wound covered with sterile 4" X 4" gauze soaked in NSS and then dry sterile dressing. P 100, BP 150/84, RR 18, T 98.6° F. Dr. McBride notified at 0930. Adhesive strips ordered and applied to wound. Pt. to be on bed rest until Dr. McBride visits at 1030. Pt. instructed to stay in bed with knees flexed and to call nurse for assistance with moving. Reviewed splinting incision with pillow during coughing or sneezing. Call bell placed within reach, and pt. demonstrated use. Pt. denies pain and is free from objective signs of discomfort. ————— *Maureen Dunlop, RN*

Infection

Infection is a relatively common complication of wound healing that should be addressed promptly.

Signs of infection

- Redness and warmth of the margins and tissue around the wound
- Fever
- Edema
- Pain (or a sudden increase in pain)
- Pus
- Increase in exudate or a change in its color
- Odor
- Discoloration of granulation tissue
- Further wound breakdown or lack of progress toward healing

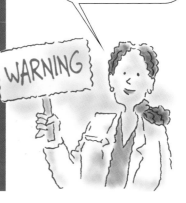

Infection can lead to cellulitis or bacterial infection that spreads to surrounding tissue. So, be alert!

WARNING

Recognizing wound infection

Clean wound

The wound here is healing properly. It's clean and has no redness, swelling, or drainage.

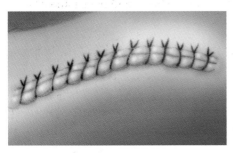

Infected wounds

These wounds show signs of infection.

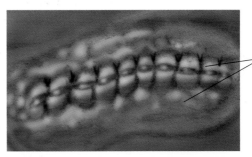

Redness and swelling along the incision line and in surrounding tissue

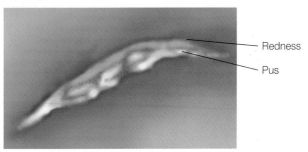

Redness

Pus

Fistulas and sinus tracts

A fistula is an abnormal passage between an organ or a vessel and another organ, vessel, or area of the skin. A sinus tract, also known as *tunneling*, is a channel that extends through part of a wound and into adjacent tissue. These complications can result in dead space and infection.

This tunnel covers a lot of territory underground. Likewise, sinus tracts are wound channels that can extend into subcutaneous tissue and muscle.

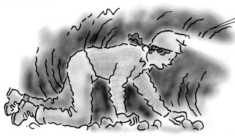

Undermining

Undermining is tissue destruction that occurs around a wound's edges, causing the skin to come away from the base of the wound (even though it may appear intact). It can develop into sinus tracts to nearby tissue.

Undermining should be carefully probed to determine how far it extends under intact skin.

Undermining is tissue destruction around the borders of a wound. It results in a wound bed that extends under the skin.

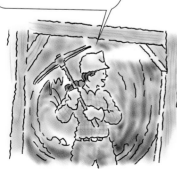

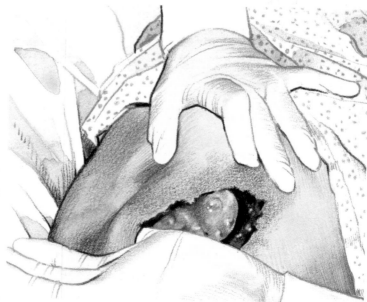

VISION QUEST

Matchmaker

Match each illustration to the proper phase of wound healing.

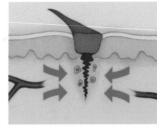

A. _____

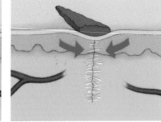

B. _____

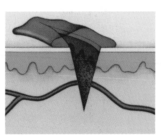

C. _____

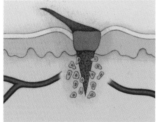

D. _____

1. Hemostasis
2. Inflammation
3. Proliferation
4. Maturation

My word!

Unscramble the names of four complications of wound healing. Then use the circled letters to answer the question posed.

Question: Which sign of failure to heal is caused by ischemia and requires wound debridement?

1. icravesitone __ __ O __ __ __ O __ __ __ __ __

2. sciencehed __ O __ __ O __ __ O __ __

3. niceifnot __ __ __ __ __ O __ __ O __

4. usaflit __ __ O __ __ __ __

Answer: __ __ __ __ __ __ __ __ __

Answers: Matchmaker 1. C, 2. D, 3. A, 4. B; My word! 1. Evisceration, 2. Dehiscence, 3. Infection, 4. Fistula; Question: Necrosis.

3
Wound assessment

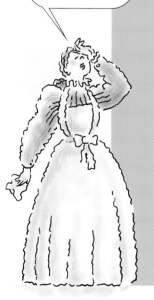

Assess my wounds? How, pray tell, can mere words describe the depth of my despair?

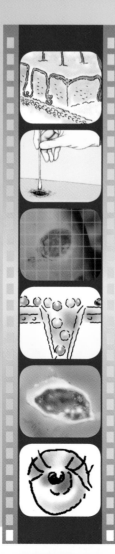

Wound classification

The words used to describe a wound must communicate the same thing to members of the health care team, insurance companies, regulators, the patient's family and, ultimately, the patient himself. The best way to classify wounds is to use the basic system described here, which focuses on three categories of fundamental characteristics:

1 Wound age

2 Wound depth

3 Wound color

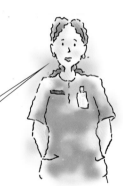

Even when the wound bed appears healthy, red, and moist, if healing fails to progress, consider the wound to be chronic.

Wound age

The first step in classifying a wound is to determine whether the wound is acute or chronic. Be careful, you can't base your determination solely on time because no set time frame specifies when an acute wound becomes chronic.

Characteristics of acute and chronic wounds

Acute	Chronic
■ New or relatively new wound	■ May develop over time
■ Occurs suddenly	■ Healing has slowed or stopped
■ Healing progresses in a timely, predictable manner	■ Typically heals by secondary intention
■ Typically heals by primary intention	■ Examples: Pressure, vascular, and diabetic ulcers
■ Examples: Surgical and traumatic wounds	

Wound depth

Wound depth can be classified as partial thickness or full thickness.

> In the case of pressure ulcers, wound depth allows you to stage the ulcer according to the classification system developed by the National Pressure Ulcer Advisory Panel. (See chapter 6, Pressure ulcers.)

Partial-thickness wound

Partial-thickness wounds involve only the epidermis or extend into the dermis but not through it.

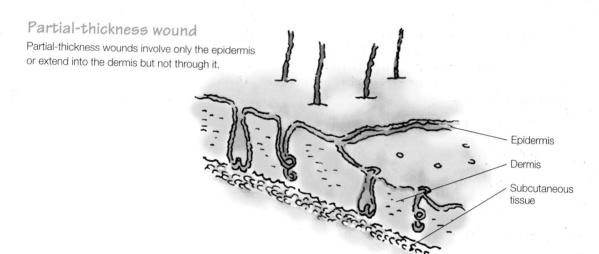

Epidermis

Dermis

Subcutaneous tissue

Full-thickness wound

Full-thickness wounds extend through the dermis into tissues beneath and may expose adipose tissue, muscle, or bone.

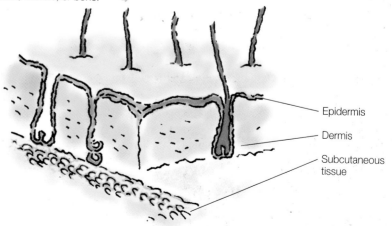

Epidermis

Dermis

Subcutaneous tissue

Measuring wound depth

To measure the depth of a wound, you'll need gloves, a cotton-tipped swab, and a disposable measuring device. This method can also be used to measure wound tunneling or undermining.

1 Put on gloves and gently insert the swab into the deepest portion of the wound.

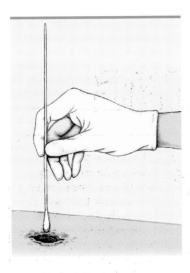

2 Grasp the swab with your fingers at the point that corresponds to the wound's margin. You can carefully mark the swab where it meets the edge of the skin.

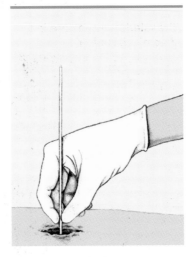

3 Remove the swab and measure the distance from your fingers or from the mark on the swab to the end of the swab to determine the depth.

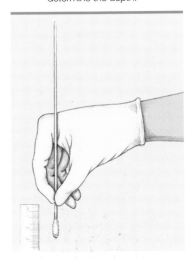

Wound color

The Red-Yellow-Black Classification System is a commonly used approach that can help you determine how well a wound is healing and develop effective wound care management plans.

Red wounds

Red indicates normal healing. When a wound begins to heal, a layer of pale pink granulation tissue covers the wound bed. As this layer thickens, it becomes beefy red.

RED WOUNDS = HEALING

Granulation tissue in an abdominal wound

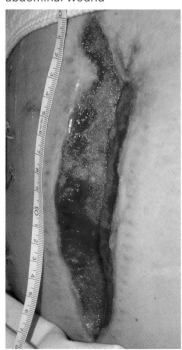

Granulation tissue base in a diabetic foot ulcer

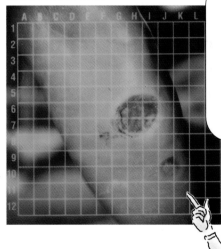

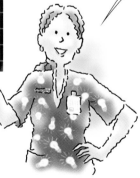

The grid in this photo allows for measuring wound area (the squares are counted and multiplied) and monitoring wound progress (the number of squares should decrease as healing progresses).

Yellow wounds

Fibrin left over from the healing process usually appears as avascular yellow slough or dead tissue on the wound base. This slough, or soft necrotic tissue, provides a medium for bacterial growth.

YELLOW WOUNDS = CAUTION

Sacral pressure ulcer with 75% of the surface area covered in yellow necrotic slough

Diabetic foot ulcer with a slough-covered base and calloused edges

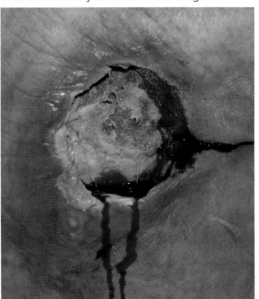

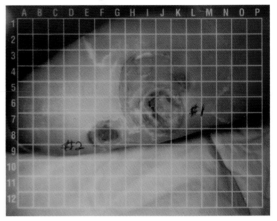

Black wounds

Black, the least healthy wound color, signals necrosis. Avascular dead tissue (known as *eschar*) slows healing and provides a site for microorganisms to proliferate.

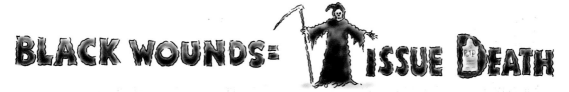

Black pressure ulcer

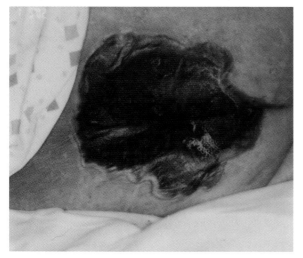

Black ischemic toe ulcers

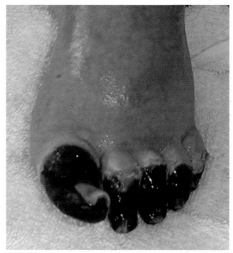

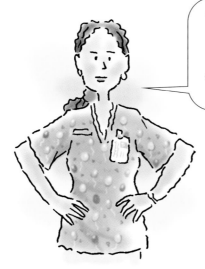

When eschar covers a wound, accurate assessment of wound depth is difficult and should be deferred until eschar is removed.

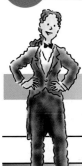

Best dressed

Tailoring wound care to wound color

Wound color	Management technique
Red	■ Cover the wound, keep it moist and clean, and protect it from trauma. ■ Use a transparent dressing (such as Tegaderm or OpSite) over a gauze dressing moistened with normal saline solution, or use a hydrogel, foam, or hydrocolloid dressing to insulate and protect the wound.
Yellow	■ Clean the wound and remove the yellow layer. ■ Cover the wound with a moisture-retentive dressing (such as a hydrogel or foam dressing or a moist gauze dressing with or without a debriding enzyme). ■ Consider hydrotherapy with whirlpool, pulsatile lavage, or ultrasonic debridement.
Black	■ Debride the wound as ordered. Use an enzyme product (such as Collagenase SANTYL), conservative sharp debridement, or hydrotherapy with whirlpool or pulsatile lavage. ■ For wounds with inadequate blood supply and uninfected heel ulcers, don't debride. Keep them clean and dry.

Classifying multicolored wounds

If you note two or even all three colors in a wound, classify the wound according to the least healthy color present. For example, if your patient's wound appears both red and yellow, classify it as a yellow wound.

Yes, I know you're mostly yellow, but for classification purposes, we're going to have to call you black.

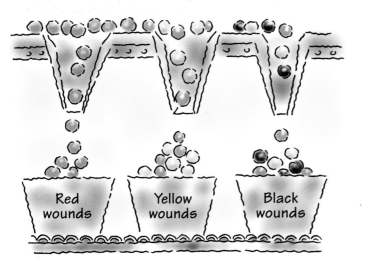

Red wounds

Yellow wounds

Black wounds

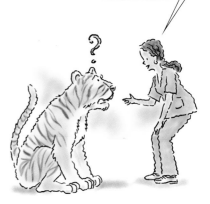

Wound terminology

Every wound has a different size, shape, and color, which can make accurate documentation challenging. However, understanding and using standard terminology can make the job easier.

Call 'em like you see 'em

When you visually examine a wound, look for the following key characteristics.

What do you see?

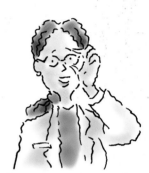

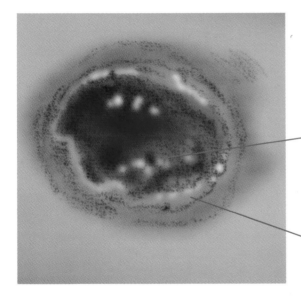

Beefy red, bumpy, shiny tissue in the base of an ulcer

- This indicates **granulation tissue**.
- As a wound heals, it develops more and more granulation tissue.

Pale or dark pink skin

- This indicates **epithelial tissue**.
- Epithelial tissue first appears at ulcer borders in full-thickness wounds and as islands around hair follicles in partial-thickness wounds.

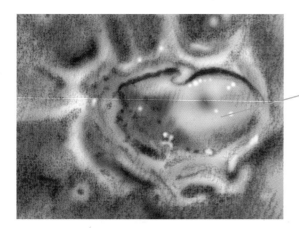

Moist yellow or gray area of tissue that's separating from viable tissue

- This is **slough** and indicates soft, necrotic tissue.
- Slough provides an ideal medium for bacterial growth.

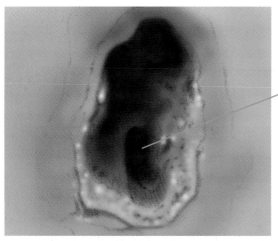

Thick, hard, leathery black tissue

- This is **eschar** and indicates dry, necrotic tissue.
- For healing to occur, necrotic tissue, drainage, and metabolic wastes must be removed.

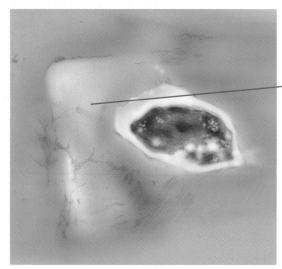

Waterlogged skin; possibly white at the wound edges

- This indicates **macerated tissue**.
- A dressing that provides too much moisture can cause maceration of surrounding skin, unless the skin is protected.
- Other common causes of maceration include wound drainage or contamination with urine or feces.

Wound drainage

A thorough wound assessment includes assessing drainage. To begin collecting information about wound drainage, inspect the dressing as it's removed and record your findings.

Drainage descriptors

Description	Color and consistency
Serous	• Clear or light yellow • Thin and watery
Sanguineous	• Red (with fresh blood) • Thin
Serosanguineous	• Pink to light red • Thin • Watery
Purulent	• Creamy yellow, green, white, or tan • Thick and opaque

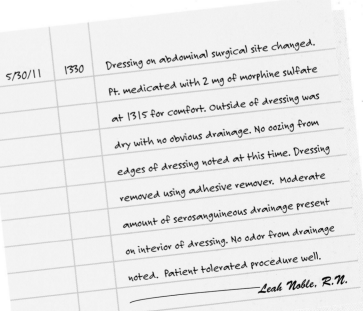

take note

Documenting wound drainage

5/30/11	1330	Dressing on abdominal surgical site changed. Pt. medicated with 2 mg of morphine sulfate at 1315 for comfort. Outside of dressing was dry with no obvious drainage. No oozing from edges of dressing noted at this time. Dressing removed using adhesive remover. Moderate amount of serosanguineous drainage present on interior of dressing. No odor from drainage noted. Patient tolerated procedure well. ———Leah Noble, R.N.

Wound measurement

When measuring a wound, you must determine its length, width, and depth. (Measuring wound depth is described on page 26.) You must also measure the surrounding areas.

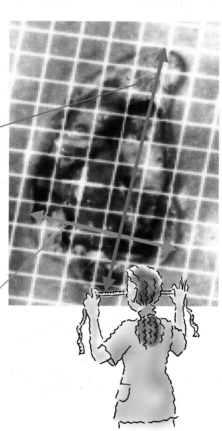

Length

- First, determine the longest distance across the open area of the wound—regardless of orientation.
- In this photo, note the line used to illustrate length.

Width

- Next, determine the longest distance across the wound at a right angle to the length.
- In this photo, note the relationship between length and width.

Surrounding areas

- Note areas of reddened, intact skin; indurated (or hard) skin; and white (macerated) skin.
- These areas are measured and recorded as surrounding erythema, induration, and maceration, not as part of the wound itself.

Measuring wound tunneling

Tunneling, also known as *undermining*, is tissue destruction that occurs around the wound perimeter underlying intact skin, causing the wound edges to pull away from the wound's base. Because tunneling may be more extensive in one part of a wound than another, measuring and documenting the location and depth of tunneling is an essential component of a wound assessment.

Probing the issue

■ Put on sterile gloves. Gently probe the wound bed and edges with your finger or a sterile cotton-tipped applicator to assess for wound tunneling.
■ Gently insert the applicator into the wound in the direction where the deepest tunneling occurs, as shown below.

Marking progress

■ Grasp the applicator where it meets the wound edge.
■ Remove the applicator, keeping your hand in place, and place it next to the measuring guide to determine the length of tunneling in centimeters, as shown below.

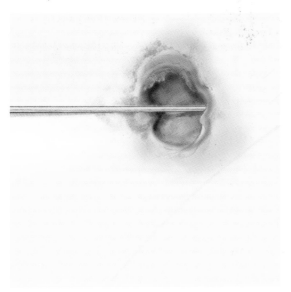

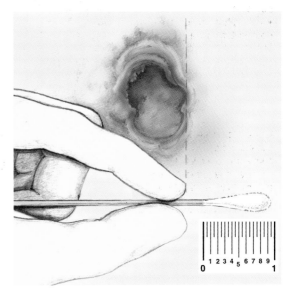

Wound documentation

Proper documentation accurately portrays the characteristics of a wound and its status in the healing process.

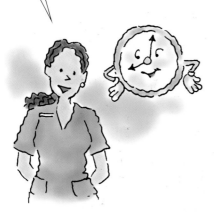

You can use the face of a clock to help document the direction of tunneling. For example, "Tunnel is 1.3 cm at 8 o'clock."

memory board

Use the mnemonic device **WOUNDD PICTURE** to help you recall and organize all of the key facts that should be included in your documentation of a wound:

Wound or ulcer location

Odor (in room or just when wound is uncovered)

Ulcer category, stage (for pressure ulcer) or classification (for diabetic ulcer), and depth (partial thickness or full thickness)

Necrotic tissue

Dimension (shape, length, width, and depth)

Drainage color, consistency, and amount (scant, moderate, or large)

Pain (when it occurs, what relieves it, patient's description, and patient's rating on scale of 0 to 10)

Induration (hard or soft surrounding tissue)

Color of wound bed (red, yellow, black, or combination)

Tunneling (length and direction—toward the patient's right, left, head, or feet)

Undermining (record length and direction, using clock references to describe)

Redness or other discoloration in surrounding skin

Edge of skin loose or tightly adhered and flat or rolled under

What's missing from this picture?

Wound photography may be a routine part of your facility's wound documentation system. Photographs can provide benchmarks for and facilitate documentation of wound healing.

Even though a picture may be "worth a thousand words," remember that your assessment skills and personal observations are still essential because many wound characteristics can't be recorded accurately— or at all—on film. For example, look at the photograph below and consider which wound characteristics you can't assess. Examples include:

- location
- depth
- tunnel measurement
- odor
- feel of surrounding tissue
- pain.

All of this information is needed if the health care team is to make sound treatment decisions.

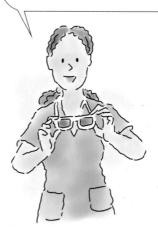

A special technology called sterophotogrammetry involves using overlapping photographs to provide a three-dimentional wound image. I guess I won't be needing these anymore then.

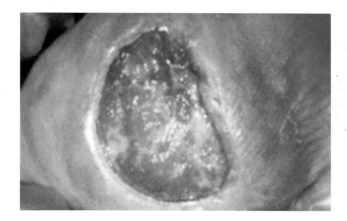

VISION QUEST

Matchmaker

Match each photo with the terminology that describes the characteristics of the wound.

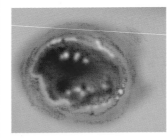

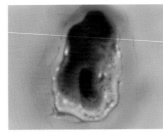

1. _____

2. _____

A. Macerated tissue
B. Granulation tissue
C. Eschar
D. Slough

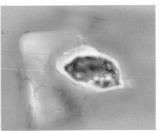

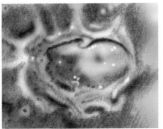

3. _____

4. _____

Show and tell

Describe the three steps used to measure wound depth that are shown here.

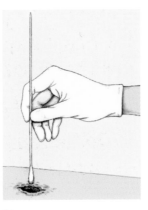

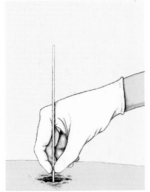

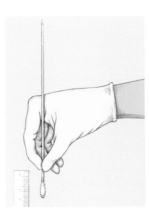

1. _____
_____
_____

2. _____
_____
_____

3. _____
_____
_____

Answers: Matchmaker 1. B, 2. C, 3. A, 4. D; Show and tell 1. Insert the swab into the deepest portion of the wound. 2. Grasp the swab at the point where it meets the wound's margin. 3. Remove the swab and measure the distance from your finger to the end of the swab.

4 Wound care procedures

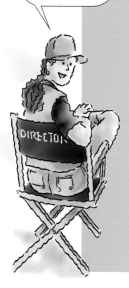

Listen up, people! We have a lot of procedures to cover before we can "wrap things up."

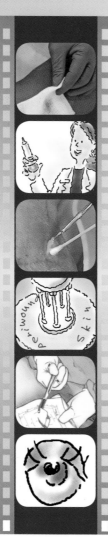

Cleaning a wound

The goal of wound cleaning is to remove debris and contaminants from the wound without damaging healthy tissue. After an initial cleaning, wounds should be cleaned as needed and before a new dressing is applied.

Step by step

As you follow these steps, be sure to observe standard precautions. Follow facility protocols regarding use of clean or sterile technique.

1 Remove the soiled dressing. Roll or lift an edge of the dressing and then gently remove it while supporting the surrounding skin. When possible, remove the dressing in the direction of hair growth.

2 Inspect the dressing and wound. Note the color, amount, and odor of drainage and necrotic debris.

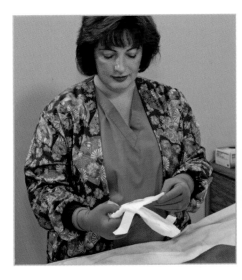

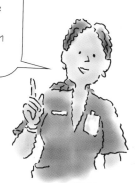

When cleaning a wound, move from the least contaminated area to the most contaminated area. Also, be sure to use a clean gauze pad for each wipe.

Cleaning techniques

To clean a linear shaped wound (such as an incision), gently wipe from top to bottom in one motion, starting directly over the wound and moving outward, as shown below.

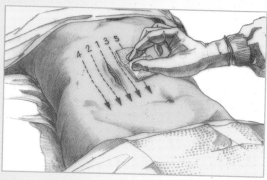

3 **Clean the wound.** Moisten gauze pads either by dipping the pads in wound cleaning solution and wringing out excess or by using a spray gun bottle to apply solution to the gauze.

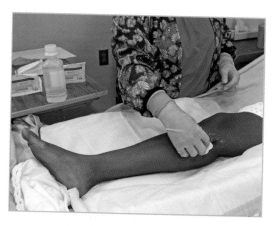

For an open wound (such as a pressure ulcer), gently wipe in concentric circles, starting directly over the wound and moving outward, as shown below.

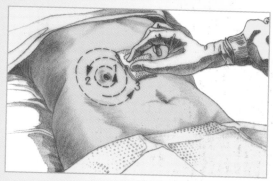

4 Dry the wound. Using the same procedure as for cleaning a wound, dry the wound using dry gauze pads.

5 Reassess the condition of the skin and wound. Note the character of the clean wound bed and surrounding skin.

Wound reassessment algorithm

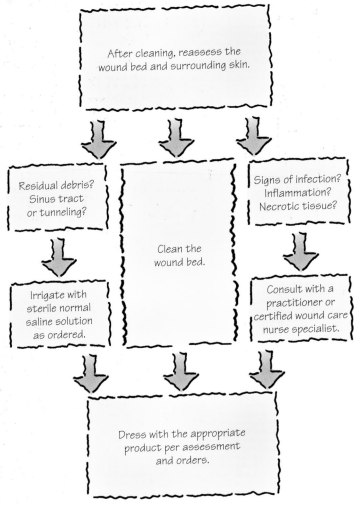

After cleaning, reassess the wound bed and surrounding skin.

Residual debris? Sinus tract or tunneling?

Clean the wound bed.

Signs of infection? Inflammation? Necrotic tissue?

Irrigate with sterile normal saline solution as ordered.

Consult with a practitioner or certified wound care nurse specialist.

Dress with the appropriate product per assessment and orders.

6 Pack or dress the wound as ordered.

Choosing a cleaning agent

The type of cleaning agent you'll use on a wound depends on the wound type and characteristics.

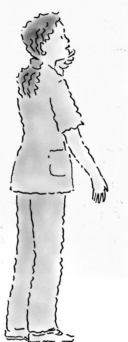

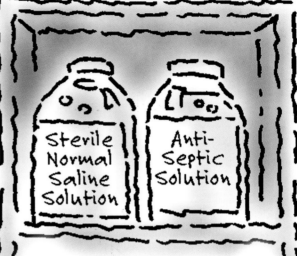

- Most commonly used cleaning agent
- Provides a moist environment
- Promotes granulation tissue formation
- Causes minimal fluid shifts in healthy adults

- Sometimes used to clean infected or newly contaminated wounds
- May damage healthy tissue and delay wound healing

> Watch for patient sensitivity to povidone-iodine.

Types of antiseptic solutions

Hydrogen peroxide	Acetic acid	Sodium hypochlorite (Dakin's solution)	Povidone-iodine	Chlorhexidine
■ Used to clean or irrigate as mechanical debridement aid ■ Promotes vasodilation through warmth of foaming action ■ Reduces inflammation ■ Commonly used half-strength ■ Avoid use in sinus tracts due to risk of air embolism	■ Used to treat *Pseudomonas* infection ■ Verify active infection by culture before use ■ 0.5% to 5% strength depending on order	■ Used to kill gram-negative bacteria per culture ■ Slightly dissolves necrotic tissue ■ Must be freshly prepared every 24 hours (solution is unstable)	■ Used to kill broad spectrum of bacteria ■ May dry and stain the surrounding skin; protect from contact ■ Toxic with prolonged use or over large areas ■ Avoid use in patients with thyroid disease	■ Used to kill gram-positive and gram-negative bacteria ■ Must be diluted

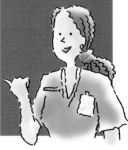

Irrigating a wound

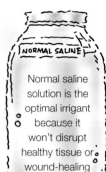

NORMAL SALINE

Normal saline solution is the optimal irrigant because it won't disrupt healthy tissue or wound-healing cells.

Irrigation serves to:
- clean tissues
- flush cell debris and drainage from an open wound
- prevent premature surface healing over an abscess pocket or infected tract.

Step by step

As you follow these steps, be sure to observe standard precautions and maintain sterile technique.

1 **Prepare the solution and equipment.** Fill the irrigating device with irrigating solution.

2 **Irrigate the entire wound thoroughly.**
Gently instill a slow, steady stream of solution into the wound (below left). Make sure the solution flows from the clean area to the dirty area of the wound to prevent contamination of clean tissue. To prevent tissue damage, don't force the needle or angiocatheter into the wound. Irrigate until you've administered the prescribed amount of solution or until the solution returns clear. Note the amount of solution administered. Keep the patient positioned to allow complete wound drainage (below right).

Devices used to irrigate a wound should provide gentle, low-pressure irrigation and may include a bulb syringe or a 35-ml piston syringe with an 18-gauge needle or angiocatheter.

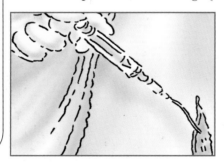

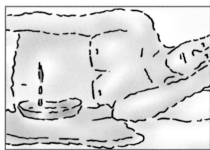

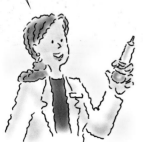

3 **Clean and dry the skin.** Use normal saline solution on the periwound skin, and then pat it dry with gauze.

4 **Pack or dress the wound as ordered.**

Packing a wound

Packing is used for mechanical debridement of a wound and to prevent surface healing before deep healing. The type of packing material used depends on the size of the wound and the amount of exudate.

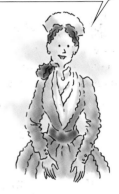

Times have changed! Cotton mesh gauze used to be the standard in packing material. Today, you have more options.

Step by step

As you follow these steps, be sure to observe standard precautions.

1 **Make sure the packing material is moist.** Use a slight amount of sterile normal saline solution if needed.

2 **Pack the wound.** Use sterile forceps and cotton-tipped applicators as needed.
 – Fluff the moist sterile packing pad or strip to unclump it.
 – Loosely but thoroughly pack the wound. Note that packing the wound too tightly can create pressure damage on the granulating cells.
 – Cover all the wound surfaces and edges.
 – Pack only in the wound bed because packing material can macerate intact tissue.

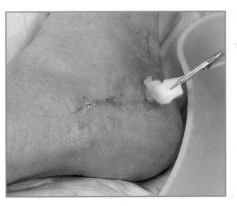
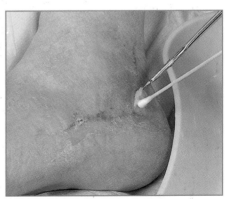

3 **Dress with dry sterile gauze.**

Dressing a wound

I'm here at the annual Wound Dressing Competition. As any fan of this competition knows, the winning dressing always provides an optimal environment in which the body can heal.

Competition is fierce. Contestants are judged on their ability to keep wounds moist, absorb drainage, conform to the wound, and be comfortable. Let's go to the competition floor.

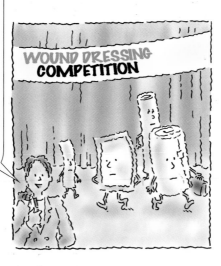

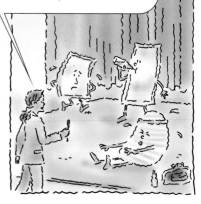

The composite dressing is taking his turn. He has scored a perfect 10 in his compulsories and is now performing his individual program. What a unique combination! Let's see how he thinks he scored.

I did my best in adhering to the surrounding skin, decreasing the need for a secondary dressing, and showing my user-friendly side. Let's hope the judges also find me cost-effective.

Can I tell it like it is? I think you've impressed the judges. We'll have to see how the other contestants perform, though.

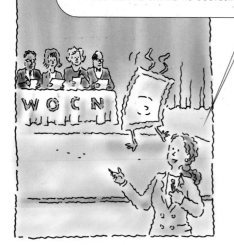

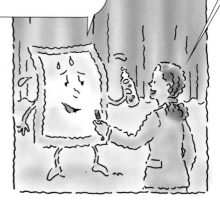

Wound dressing algorithm

Use nonadherent dressing held with stretch gauze or netting.

Fragile & thin

No special care is needed.

Has a rash

Better check with practitioner.

Healthy

To determine the appropriate dressing for your patient's wound, start by assessing the periwound skin.

Warm, inflamed, & sore

UNBROKEN and...

Use protective film barrier

Check with practitioner

Has a yeast infection

periwound skin

Red

Use hydrocolloid wafer, paste, or powder.

Has lost the top layer of skin

BROKEN and...

Macerated

Change primary dressing.

Use petroleum-based ointment, zinc oxide, or barrier film on edges.

Both

Fragile and weeping

Hold with nonadherent dressing with stretch gauze or netting.

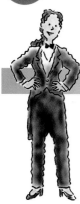

Best dressed

Step-by-step wound dressing

Regardless of the dressing or topical agent you use, follow your facility's protocol or the manufacturer's instructions for applying the wound dressing.

Type of dressing	Application method
Alginate	▪ Apply the dressing to the wound surface. ▪ Cover the area with a secondary dressing (such as gauze pads or transparent film), as ordered. ▪ Secure the dressing with tape or elastic netting. ▪ If the wound is heavily draining, change the dressing once or twice daily for the first 3 to 5 days. As drainage decreases, change the dressing less frequently—every 2 to 4 days or as ordered. When the drainage stops or the wound bed looks dry, stop using alginate dressings.
Foam	▪ Gently lay the dressing over the wound. ▪ Use tape, elastic netting, or gauze to hold the dressing in place. ▪ Change the dressing when the foam no longer absorbs exudate.
Hydrocolloid	▪ Choose a clean, dry, presized dressing or cut one to overlap the wound by about 1″ (2.5 cm). ▪ Remove the dressing from its package. ▪ Pull the release paper from the adherent side of the dressing. ▪ Apply the dressing to the wound, carefully smoothing out wrinkles and avoiding stretching the dressing. ▪ Hold the dressing in place with your hand (the warmth from your hand will mold the dressing to the skin). ▶ ▪ If the dressing's edges need to be secured with tape, apply a skin sealant to the intact skin around the wound. After the area dries, tape the dressing to the skin. The sealant protects the skin from tape burns and skin stripping and promotes tape adherence. Avoid using tension or pressure when you apply the tape. ▪ Change the dressing every 2 to 7 days as necessary; change it immediately if the patient complains of pain, the dressing no longer adheres, or leakage occurs.

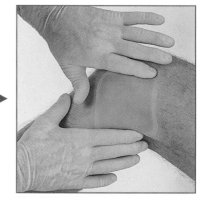

Type of dressing	Application method	
Hydrogel	▪ Apply a moderate amount of gel to the wound bed. ▪ Cover the area with a secondary dressing (gauze, transparent film, or foam). ▪ Change the dressing daily or as needed to keep the wound bed moist. ▪ If the dressing you select comes in sheet form, cut the dressing to overlap the wound by 1″ (2.5 cm); then apply as you would a hydrocolloid dressing. *Note:* Hydrogel dressings also come as prepackaged, saturated gauze for wounds with cavities that require "dead space" to be filled. Follow the manufacturer's directions to apply these dressings.	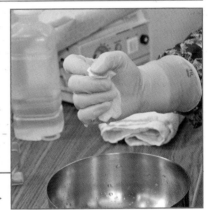
Moist saline gauze	▪ Moisten the dressing with normal saline solution. ▪ Wring out excess fluid. ▪ Gently place the dressing onto the wound surface, molding the moist gauze around the wound. ▪ To separate surfaces within the wound, gently guide the gauze between opposing wound surfaces. To avoid damage to tissues, don't pack the gauze tightly. ▪ Apply a sealant or barrier to protect the surrounding skin from moisture. ▪ Change the dressing frequently enough to keep the wound moist.	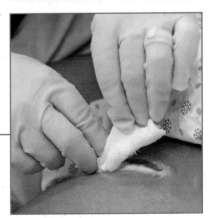
Transparent	▪ Select a dressing to overlap the wound by 1″ to 2″ (2.5 to 5 cm). ▪ Gently lay the dressing over the wound; avoid wrinkling the dressing. To prevent shearing force, don't stretch the dressing over the wound. Press firmly on the edges of the dressing to promote adherence. ▪ Change the dressing every 3 to 5 days, depending on the amount of drainage. If the seal is no longer secure, change the dressing.	

Applying a wound pouch

A wound with copious drainage may need to have a pouch applied. A wound pouch collects drainage and helps protect the surrounding skin.

Step by step

When applying a wound pouch, wear a gown and a face shield or mask and goggles in case the drainage splashes. Be sure to follow standard precautions when performing the following steps.

1 **Measure the wound.** Use a disposable measuring tape to obtain the wound's length and width.

3 **Apply a skin protectant as needed.** Note that some protectants are incorporated within the wafer and also provide adhesion.

2 **Cut an opening in the wafer.** The opening should be ³⁄₈″ (1 cm) larger than the wound (as shown below).

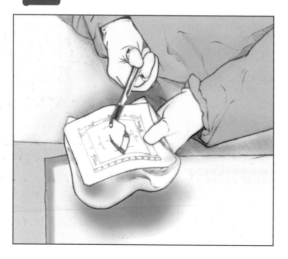

5 Empty the pouch as needed. Insert the bottom half of the pouch into a graduated biohazard container, and open the drainage port (as shown below).
– Note the color, consistency, odor, and amount of fluid.
– If ordered, obtain a culture specimen and immediately send it to the laboratory.
– Wipe the bottom of the pouch and the drainage port with a gauze pad to remove drainage, which could irritate the patient's skin or cause an odor.
– Reseal the port.

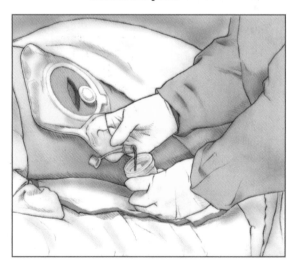

4 Press the contoured pouch opening around the wound. Start at the lowest edge of the wound to catch any drainage (as shown below).
– Make sure the drainage port at the bottom of the pouch is closed firmly to prevent leaks.
– Be gentle but firm to avoid causing pain; offer to hold the wafer in place while the patient presses, if preferred.

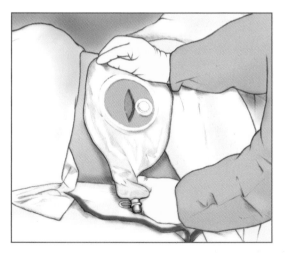

6 Change the pouch as needed. Only change the pouch if it leaks or fails to adhere as more frequent changes may irritate the patient's skin.

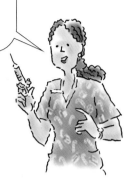

The surface swab technique obtains bacteria colonized only on the wound's surface. For a more accurate culture, needle aspiration of fluid or punch tissue biopsy should be used.

Collecting a wound culture

Infected wounds (those with heavy bacterial or fungal overgrowth) are unable to properly heal. Cultures can help to determine the involved organism and guide treatment. One common wound culture collection method is the surface swab technique. Other methods, including syringe aspiration and punch tissue biopsy, are performed by advanced practice nurses and physicians.

Step by step

When obtaining a wound culture, follow standard precautions and maintain sterile technique throughout each of these steps.

1 Inspect and irrigate. After inspecting the wound, thoroughly irrigate it with sterile saline solution.

2 Rotate a sterile swab along all areas of the wound. Gently twist the calcium alginate or rayon swab (not cotton-tipped) on the sides and base of the wound, crossing the entire surface of the wound. To ensure all possible areas of infection have been swabbed, use the 10-point coverage system.

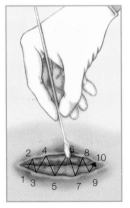

3 Place the swab in the appropriate culture medium. If the wound is open and has viable tissue, immediately place the swab in an aerobic culture tube. If the wound has necrotic tissue or sinus tracts, obtain both an aerobic and an anaerobic culture.

4 Label the culture tube. Include the patient's name, the date and time, the source location of the specimen, and any antibiotics the patient is taking. Immediately send the tube to the laboratory.

Collecting an anaerobic specimen

Because most anaerobes die when exposed to oxygen, they must be transported in tubes filled with carbon dioxide or nitrogen. Before specimen collection, the small inner tube containing the swab is held in place with a rubber stopper.

After collecting the specimen, quickly replace the swab in the inner tube and depress the plunger to separate the inner tube from the stopper. The swab is forced into the larger tube, exposing the specimen to a carbon dioxide–rich environment.

Before   After

Debriding a wound

Debridement is the removal of necrotic (dead) tissue and debris (such as eschar) from a wound. When combined with optimal nutrition, circulation, mobility, and attitude toward healing, debridement can help to promote wound healing.

Just as there's more than one way to shoot a scene, there's more than one way to debride a wound.

Understanding debridement methods

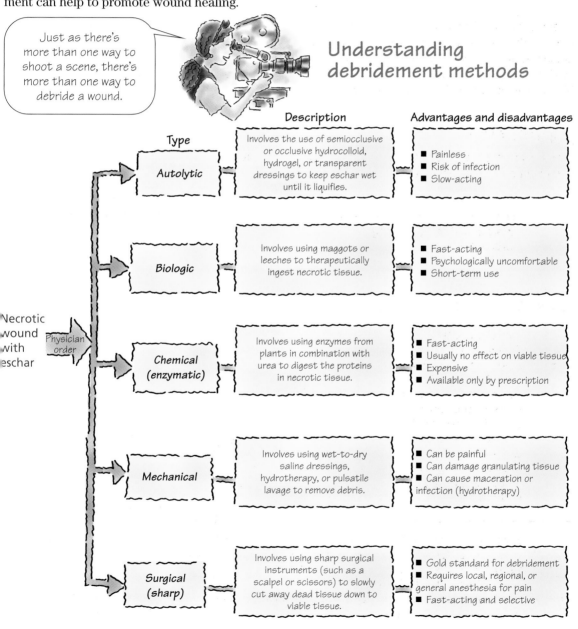

Type	Description	Advantages and disadvantages
Autolytic	Involves the use of semiocclusive or occlusive hydrocolloid, hydrogel, or transparent dressings to keep eschar wet until it liquifies.	■ Painless ■ Risk of infection ■ Slow-acting
Biologic	Involves using maggots or leeches to therapeutically ingest necrotic tissue.	■ Fast-acting ■ Psychologically uncomfortable ■ Short-term use
Chemical (enzymatic)	Involves using enzymes from plants in combination with urea to digest the proteins in necrotic tissue.	■ Fast-acting ■ Usually no effect on viable tissue ■ Expensive ■ Available only by prescription
Mechanical	Involves using wet-to-dry saline dressings, hydrotherapy, or pulsatile lavage to remove debris.	■ Can be painful ■ Can damage granulating tissue ■ Can cause maceration or infection (hydrotherapy)
Surgical (sharp)	Involves using sharp surgical instruments (such as a scalpel or scissors) to slowly cut away dead tissue down to viable tissue.	■ Gold standard for debridement ■ Requires local, regional, or general anesthesia for pain ■ Fast-acting and selective

Necrotic wound with eschar → Physician order →

Assisting in sharp debridement

Sharp debridement helps to create a blood-rich, uninfected wound surface in which granulation can occur. Advanced practice nurses with specific training in this care can remove tissue that's dead or loose (has a clearly visible line where viable tissue begins). However, only a surgeon can debride wounds that cover very large areas, are deep and very close to vital structures, or whose edges can't be readily distinguished from viable tissues. General or regional anesthesia is required for this procedure.

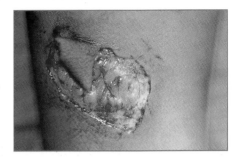

Nonviable tissue

Step by step

Follow standard precautions and maintain a sterile field and sterile technique when assisting with sharp debridement.

1 Administer an analgesic, as ordered. Give an oral drug 20 minutes before debridement, or an I.V. analgesic immediately before the procedure.

3 Apply pressure to bleeding tissues. If bleeding occurs, apply gentle pressure with sterile 4″ × 4″ gauze pads.

2 Assist the practitioner as needed. Provide assistance as the practitioner lifts the edges of eschar, holds necrotic tissue taut with sterile forceps, and cuts dead tissue from the wound. Irrigate the wound as necessary.

4 Treat and dress the site as ordered. Apply topical medications and replace and secure the dressing, as ordered.

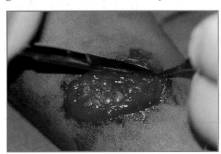

Healthy tissue

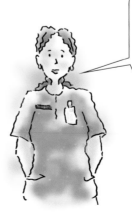

In debridement, dead tissue is removed, which exposes healthy tissue and increases the size of the wound.

Understanding biologic debridement

Maggot therapy

Maggot therapy is a type of biological therapy in which live, sterilized, medicinal *Lucilia sericata* (green bottle fly) maggots are placed in a wound every 2 to 3 days, either directly or in a saclike device. The maggots secrete a proteinase enzyme that helps degrade necrotic tissue and digest bacteria, which promotes healing in wounds with resistant microorganism strains. The maggots also stimulate formation of granulation tissue. Although cost-effective, this treatment can be painful.

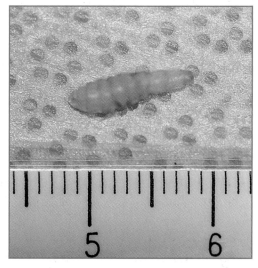

Maggot larva

Steps

- Clean the treatment area with normal saline solution.
- Place 5 to 10 sterile maggots per square centimeter of the wound, carefully counting the number of maggots you place.
- Immediately cover the wound with an absorbent dressing, according to facility protocol.
- Check the dressing every 6 hours for drainage, and change as needed.
- Remove the maggots after therapy, carefully counting to ensure that all of the maggots have been retrieved.

Contraindications

- Patients with life-threatening wounds
- Patients who would suffer psychological stress from the therapy
- Patients with bleeding abnormalities
- Patients with deep-tracking wounds

Leech therapy

In leech therapy, which is sometimes used after reattachment surgery and transplantation surgery, medical leeches (*Hirudo medicinalis*) are applied to wounds to effectively:

- relieve venous congestion
- create a puncture that bleeds
- anesthetize the wound
- prevent blood clotting
- dilate vessels to increase blood flow.

Leech therapy works because leech saliva contains hirudin, a thrombin inhibitor; hyaluronidase, which helps spread the saliva and has antibiotic properties; a histamine-like vasodilator to promote local bleeding; and a local anesthetic.

Steps

- Wash the area with soap and water and then rinse it with distilled, nonchlorinated water.
- While wearing gloves, attach the leech, directing the head toward the therapy site.
- Cover the treatment area with gauze to prevent the leech from migrating to another site.
- Monitor the site every 15 minutes.
- After therapy, remove the leech by placing a small amount of alcohol, saline solution, or vinegar on a pad or a cotton swab and stroking the head of the leech until it detaches. *Note:* Do not pull the leech.

Leech anatomy

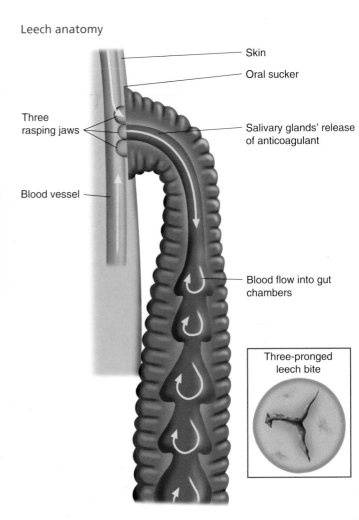

Skin

Oral sucker

Three rasping jaws

Salivary glands' release of anticoagulant

Blood vessel

Blood flow into gut chambers

Three-pronged leech bite

Documenting wound care

Documentation checklist

When documenting wound care, be sure to include:

- ☑ date, time, and type of wound care performed
- ☑ amount of soiled dressing and packing removed
- ☑ type, color, consistency, and amount of drainage
- ☑ wound appearance (size, condition of margins, presence of necrotic tissue)
- ☑ presence of odor
- ☑ presence and location of drains
- ☑ additional procedures, such as irrigation, packing, or application of a topical medication
- ☑ type and amount of new dressing or pouch applied
- ☑ patient's tolerance of the procedure.

Document special or detailed wound care instructions and pain management steps on the care plan. Also record the amount of drainage on the intake and output sheet.

take note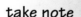

Documenting wound care

05/12/11	1430	Dressing removed from abdominal incision. 2-cm round area of serosanguineous drainage noted on dressing. No odor noted. Incision well approximated except for 1.5-cm area at distal end of incision. Wound culture obtained and sent to lab. Incision cleaned with sterile NSS and sterile dressing applied. Pt. tolerated procedure well.
		———— David Stevens, RN

VISION QUEST

Matchmaker

Match the wound cleaning technique shown with the proper wound type for which it's used.

1.

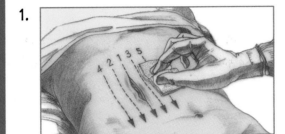

A. Circular wound
B. Linear wound

2.

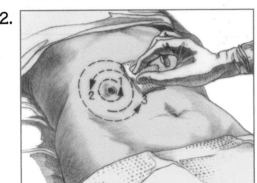

Show and tell

State which wound care procedure is illustrated here and explain why this method is used.

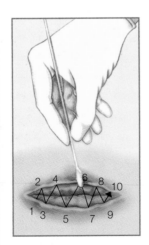

_____
_____
_____
_____
_____

Answers: Matchmaker 1. B, 2. A; Show and tell This illustration shows swab culturing using the 10-point method. The 10-point method is used to ensure all possible areas of infection have been swabbed.

5
Acute wounds

I love a script with burning passions, burning desires, and even burning buildings. But skin burns? Ouch. That's a different story entirely.

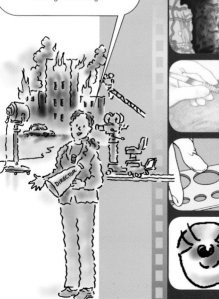

Burns

Burns are tissue injuries that result from contact with thermal, chemical, or electrical sources or from friction or exposure to the sun. They can cause cellular skin damage and a systemic response that leads to altered body function. A major burn affects every body system and organ, usually requiring painful treatment and a long period of rehabilitation.

Types of burns

First-degree

A first-degree burn causes localized injury or destruction to the skin's epidermis by direct contact (such as a chemical spill) or indirect contact (such as sunlight).

Although a first-degree burn isn't life-threatening and doesn't disrupt the barrier function of the skin, it still hurts!

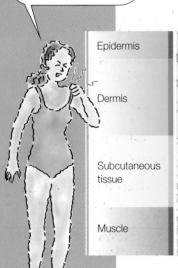

Epidermis

Dermis

Subcutaneous tissue

Muscle

Signs and symptoms

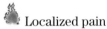

Localized pain

Localized edema

Erythema (usually without blisters)

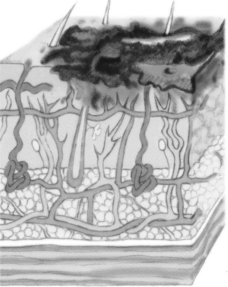

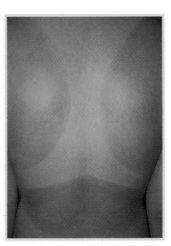

Second-degree

Second-degree burns are subclassified as either **SUPERFICIAL** partial-thickness burns or **DEEP** partial-thickness burns.

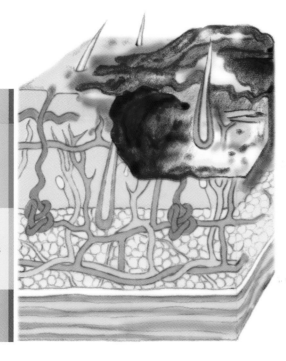

Epidermis

Dermis

Subcutaneous tissue

Muscle

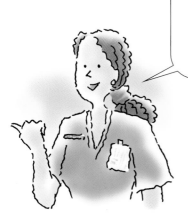

This first-degree burn resulted from sunburn. Notice the localized erythema and absence of blisters characteristic of first-degree burns.

In **SUPERFICIAL** partial-thickness burns:

🔥 epidermis and some dermis are destroyed

🔥 thin-walled, fluid-filled blisters develop within minutes of the injury

🔥 nerve endings become exposed to the air as blisters break

🔥 pain and tactile response remain intact

🔥 barrier function of the skin is lost.

In **DEEP** partial-thickness burns:

🔥 epidermis and dermis are involved

🔥 blisters develop

🔥 mild-to-moderate edema and pain occur

🔥 damaged area may have a white, waxy appearance

🔥 hair follicles remain intact, so hair can regrow

🔥 sensory neurons undergo extensive destruction.

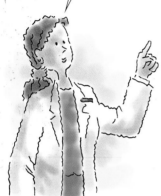

This photo shows a child with a superficial partial-thickness sunburn. Note the thin-walled, fluid-filled blisters.

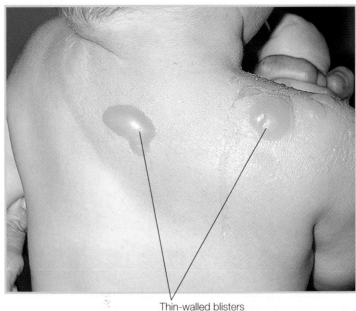

Thin-walled blisters

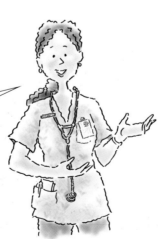

Here's another example of a superficial partial-thickness burn.

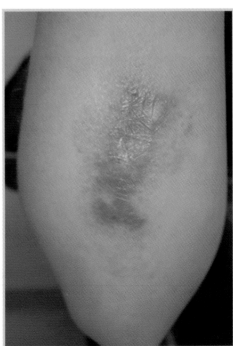

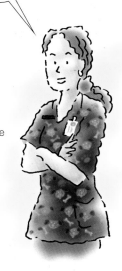

This photo shows a deep partial-thickness burn. Note the white, waxy appearance. In this instance, the large bullae will most likely be ruptured.

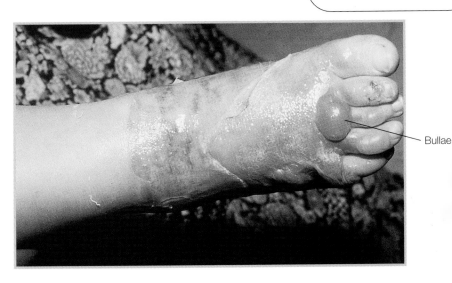

Bullae

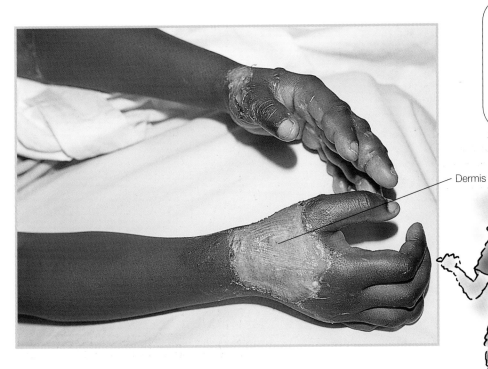

You can easily see the dermis in this deep partial-thickness burn.

Dermis

Third-degree

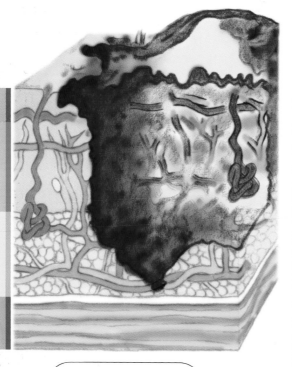

Epidermis

Dermis

Subcutaneous
tissue

Muscle

Also known as *full-thickness burns*, these burns:

🔥 extend through the epidermis and dermis and into the subcutaneous tissue layer

🔥 may involve muscle, bone, and interstitial tissues

🔥 may have a white, brown, or black leathery appearance without blisters

🔥 may reveal thrombosed vessels (due to destruction of skin elasticity)

🔥 cause fluids and protein to shift from capillary to interstitial spaces within hours, causing edema

🔥 trigger an immediate immunologic response, making burn wound sepsis a potential threat.

A third-degree burn results in an increased calorie demand, which increases the patient's metabolic rate.

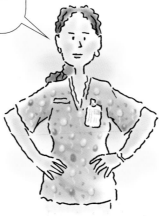

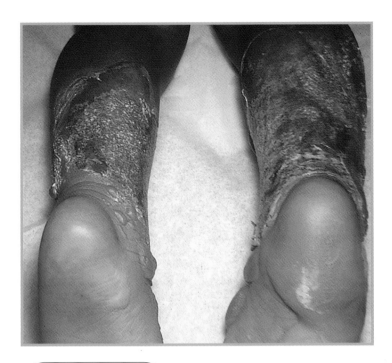

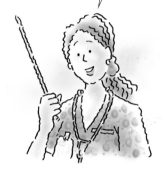

The full-thickness burns shown in this photo resulted from being scalded in a bathtub.

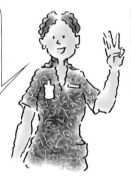

The black, leathery skin and absence of blisters over this hand and wrist are characteristic of third-degree burns.

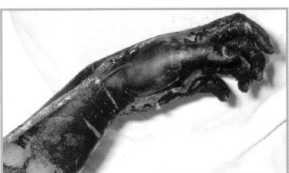

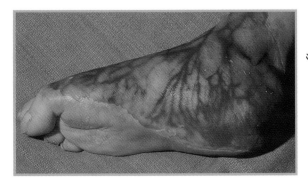

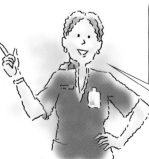

Note the thrombosed blood vessels visible in this third-degree burn of the foot.

Electrical burns

Electrical burns usually result from contact with faulty electrical wiring and cords or high-voltage power lines.

Cross-section of skin with electrical burn

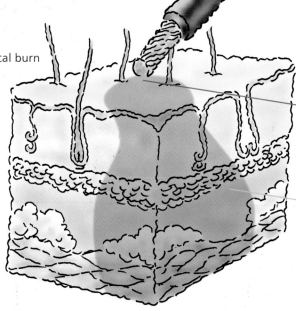

Epidermis

Dermis

Subcutaneous tissue

Muscle

At the site of electrical contact, the injury may appear silver-colored, with a raised or charred area.

Tissue damage from electrical burns is difficult to assess because internal damage along the conduction pathway is commonly greater than the surface burn indicates.

The person in this photo tried to stop a fall from a ladder by grasping a high-voltage electrical line, resulting in electrocution and an electrical burn.

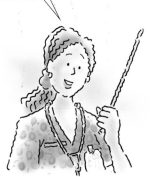

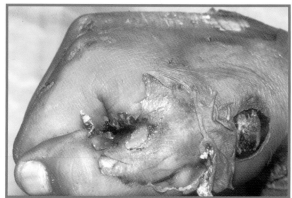

Estimating the extent of burns

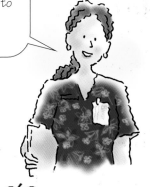

Because BSA varies with age, you'll use the Rule of Nines to estimate the extent of an adult patient's burns and the Lund-Browder classification to estimate the extent of an infant's or a child's burns.

Rule of Nines

You can quickly estimate the extent of an adult patient's burn by using the Rule of Nines. This method quantifies body surface area (BSA) in multiples of nine, giving the method its name.

To use this method, mentally assess your patient's burns according the body charts below. Add the corresponding percentages for each body section burned. Use the total—a rough estimate of the extent of the burn—to calculate initial fluid replacement needs.

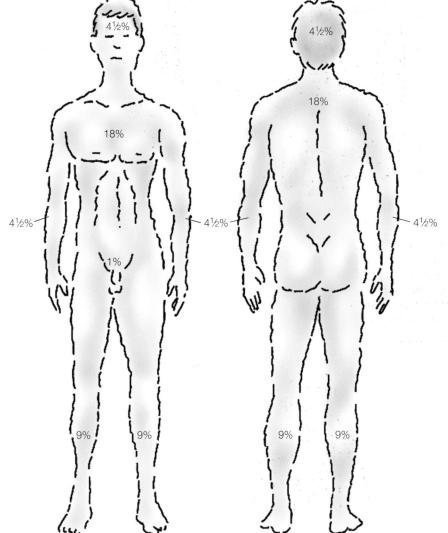

Lund-Browder classification

The Rule of Nines isn't accurate for infants or children because their body shapes, and therefore BSA, differ from those of adults. For example, an infant's head accounts for about 17% of total BSA, compared with 7% for an adult. Instead, use the Lund-Browder classification (shown below) to determine burn size for infants and children.

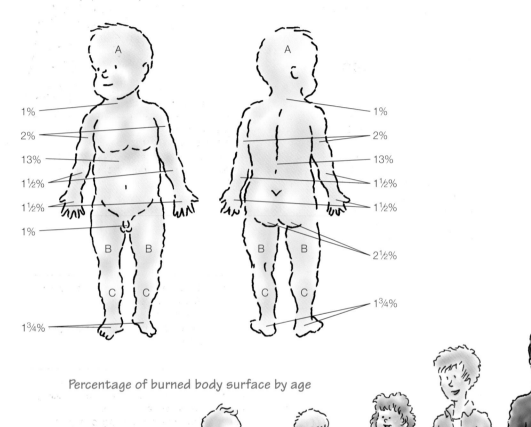

Percentage of burned body surface by age

	At birth	0 to 1 year	1 to 4 years	5 to 9 years	10 to 15 years	Adult
A: Half of head	9 1/2%	8 1/2%	6 1/2%	5 1/2%	4 1/2%	3 1/2%
B: Half of one thigh	2 3/4%	3 1/4%	4%	4 1/4%	4 1/2%	4 3/4%
C: Half of one leg	2 1/2%	2 1/2%	2 1/4%	3%	3 1/4%	3 1/2%

Biological burn dressings

Biological dressings provide a temporary protective covering for burn wounds and clean granulation tissue. They also temporarily secure fresh skin grafts and protect graft donor sites.

> In addition to stimulating new skin growth, biological dressings act like normal skin: They reduce heat loss, block infection, and minimize fluid, electrolyte, and protein losses.

Comparing biological dressings

Type	Description and uses	Nursing considerations
Cadaver (organic, homograft)	■ Obtained at autopsy up to 24 hours after death ■ Applied in the operating room or at the bedside to debrided, untidy wounds ■ Available as fresh cryopreserved homografts in tissue banks nationwide ■ Provides protection, especially to granulation tissue after escharotomy ■ May be used in some patients as a test graft for autografting ■ Covers excised wounds immediately	■ Observe for exudate. ■ Watch for signs of rejection. ■ Keep in mind that the gauze dressing may be removed every 8 hours to observe the graft.
Pigskin (organic, heterograft or xenograft)	■ Applied in the operating room or at the bedside ■ Comes fresh or frozen in rolls or sheets ■ Can cover and protect debrided, untidy wounds, mesh autografts, clean (eschar-free) partial-thickness burns, and exposed tendons	■ Reconstitute frozen form with normal saline solution 30 minutes before use. ■ Watch for signs of rejection. ■ Cover with gauze dressing or leave exposed to air, as ordered.
Amniotic membrane (organic, homograft)	■ Available from the obstetric department ■ Must be sterile and come from an uncomplicated birth; serologic tests must be done ■ Bacteriostatic condition doesn't require antimicrobials ■ May be used to protect partial-thickness burns or (temporarily) granulation tissue before autografting ■ Applied by the physician to clean wounds only	■ Change the membrane every 48 hours. ■ Cover the membrane with a gauze dressing or leave it exposed, as ordered. ■ If you apply a gauze dressing, change it every 48 hours.
Biobrane (biosynthetic membrane)	■ Comes in sterile, prepackaged sheets in various sizes and in glove form for hand burns ■ Used to cover donor graft sites, superficial partial-thickness burns, debrided wounds awaiting autograft, and meshed autografts ■ Provides significant pain relief ■ Applied by the nurse	■ Leave the membrane in place for 3 to 14 days, possibly longer. ■ Don't use this dressing for preparing a granulation bed for subsequent autografting.

Keep in mind that a patient who has received an autograft requires care for two wounds: one at the graft site and one at the donor site.

Skin grafts

Skin grafting consists of taking healthy tissue—from either the patient (autograft) or a donor (allograft)—and applying it to an area damaged by burns, traumatic injury, or surgery.

Types of skin grafts

A burn patient may receive split-thickness grafts, full-thickness grafts, or both.

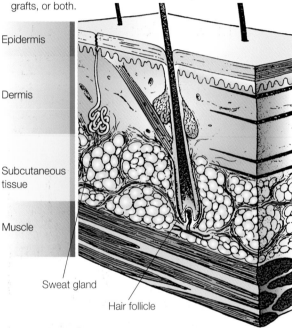

Epidermis

Dermis

Subcutaneous tissue

Muscle

Sweat gland

Hair follicle

Split-thickness skin graft

Thin 0.01″
Medium 0.02″
Thick 0.035″

Full-thickness skin graft

0.04″

Split-thickness grafts

- Include the epidermis and part of the dermis
- Commonly used to cover open burns
- May be applied as a sheet (usually on the face or neck for cosmetic purposes)
- May also be applied as a mesh (usually on extensive full-thickness burns)

Full-thickness skin grafts

- Include the epidermis and the entire dermis
- Contain hair follicles, sweat glands, and sebaceous glands
- Usually used for small deep burns

Keys to a successful skin graft

✔ Clean wound granulation with adequate vascularization

✔ Complete contact of the graft with the wound bed

✔ Maintenance of sterile technique to prevent infection

✔ Adequate graft immobilization

✔ Skilled care

Common donor skin graft sites

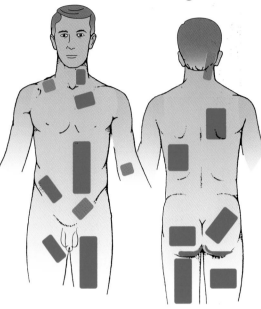

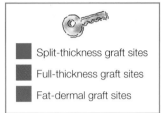

Split-thickness graft sites

Full-thickness graft sites

Fat-dermal graft sites

Caring for a donor graft site

In autografting, tissue is removed from the patient's body using a dermatome, an instrument that cuts uniform, split-thickness skin portions (shown below). Consequently, the donor site is a partial-thickness wound, which may bleed, drain, and cause pain. Depending on the graft's thickness, tissue may be obtained from the donor site again in as few as 10 days.

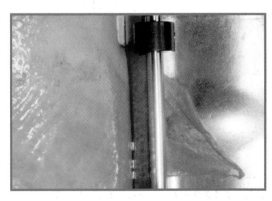

The donor site needs scrupulous care to prevent infection, which could cause the site to become a full-thickness wound.

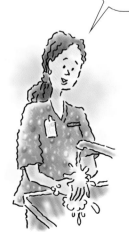

Usually, a moisture vapor–permeable dressing or Xeroflo gauze is applied postoperatively to protect new epithelial proliferation.

Dressing the wound

■ Wash your hands and put on sterile gloves.
■ Remove the outer gauze dressings within 24 hours. Inspect the Xeroflo gauze dressing for signs of infection; then leave it open to the air to speed drying and healing.
■ Leave small amounts of fluid accumulation alone. Using sterile technique, aspirate larger amounts through the dressing with a small-gauge needle and syringe.
■ Apply a lanolin-based cream daily to completely healed donor sites to keep skin tissue pliable and to remove crusts.

Evacuating fluid from a sheet graft

When small pockets of fluid (called *blebs*) accumulate beneath a sheet graft, a physician will need to evacuate the fluid using a sterile scalpel and sterile cotton-tipped applicators. Be prepared to assist, as needed.

1   The physician will carefully perforate the center of the bleb with the scalpel.

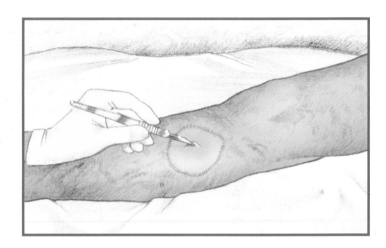

2   Then he'll gently express the fluid with the cotton-tipped applicators.

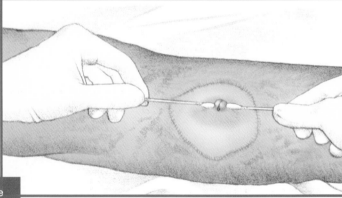

! Fluid should never be expressed by rolling the bleb to the edge of the graft. This disturbs healing in other areas.

Understanding compartment syndrome

In compartment syndrome, edema or bleeding increases pressure within a muscle compartment (arm or leg) to the point that circulation (both arterial inflow and venous outflow) to muscles and nerves within the compartment is impaired. It can occur as a result of burns, direct injury and pressure, fractures, and snake envenomation. This condition is limb-threatening and requires immediate intervention.

Symptoms

- Intense, deep, throbbing pain that doesn't improve with analgesia
- Numbness and tingling distal to the affected muscle
- Absent peripheral pulses in the affected extremity
- Pallor or mottling of the affected area
- Decreased movement, muscle strength, and sensation in the affected extremity

Treatments

- Positioning of the affected extremity at heart level
- Removal of constrictive clothing and dressings
- Analgesics
- Neurovascular status monitoring to detect changes in circulation and nerve function
- Intracompartmental pressure monitoring and Doppler ultrasound to assess blood flow
- Emergency fasciotomy to allow muscle to expand and decrease compartment pressure

Normal calf

Tibia
Muscle compartments
Fibula

Calf with compartment syndrome

Edematous muscle compartments

Compressed nerves and blood vessels

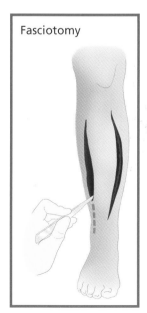

Fasciotomy

Surgical wounds

Never remove a surgical dressing without an order. Some dressings put pressure on the wound; others keep skin grafts intact.

Acute surgical wounds are uncomplicated breaks in the skin that result from surgery. In an otherwise healthy individual, these types of wounds typically heal without incident.

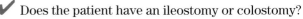

Assessment

First check the outside...

What is this? Some type of investigation?

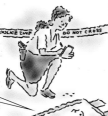
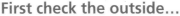

✔ Is the dressing stained?
 – Estimate drainage quantity.
 – Note its color, consistency, and odor.

✔ Does the patient have a drainage device?
 – Record the amount of drainage.
 – Note the color of the drainage.
 – Ensure that the device is patent, secure, and free from kinks.

✔ Does the patient have an ileostomy or colostomy?
 – Describe its output.
 – Monitor for signs of infection.

Just good surgical sleuthing, sir.

...then go under cover

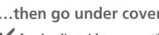
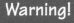

✔ Is a healing ridge present?
 – Are there signs and symptoms of infection, such as redness, warmth, and edema along the incision line and in the surrounding area; localized pain and tenderness; fever; pus or exudate from the incision; separation of suture line?

Definition: Healing ridge

Palpable ridge that forms on each side of the wound during normal wound healing. It results from a buildup of collagen fibers, which begins to form during the inflammatory phase of wound healing and peaks during the proliferation phase (approximately 5 to 9 days postoperatively). Ridges typically fail to develop because of mechanical strain on the wound.

Warning!

Wound infection is the most common surgical wound complication and the second most common infection type that occurs during hospitalization.

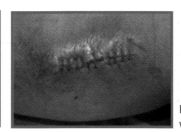

Postoperative leg wound infection

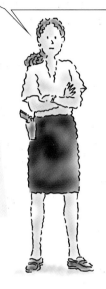

What to teach your patient about surgical wound care

☑ Signs and symptoms of wound infection to report immediately

☑ Procedure for taking an accurate temperature reading

☑ Proper wound care, such as keeping the incision clean and dry, proper hand-washing technique, and supplies and methods used to clean the wound

☑ Wound dressings, including the type, places to obtain them, and proper application

☑ Types and levels of permissible activity, such as lifting restrictions (if applicable), restrictions on bathing, and expectations for returning to work

☑ Follow-up appointments

> Being a good surgical sleuth means never going it alone. Train the patient to care for his wound and to monitor healing.

Wound closure

The severity of a wound determines the type of material used to close it.

Adhesive closures

Adhesive closures, such as Steri-Strips or butterfly closures, may be used to close small wounds with scant drainage or to provide continued reinforcement after suture or staple removal.

Steri-Strips

Steri-Strips are thin strips of sterile, nonwoven tape. They're a primary means of holding a wound closed after suture removal.

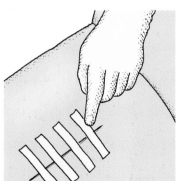

Butterfly closures

Butterfly closures consist of two sterile, waterproof adhesive strips linked by a narrow, nonadhesive "bridge." They're used to hold small wounds closed to promote healing after suture removal.

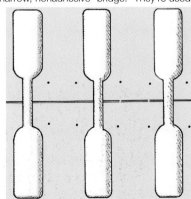

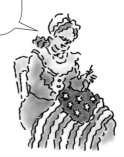

I should know. Not every job calls for the same stitch.

Suture methods

Surgeons usually use sutures. If cosmetic results aren't an issue, the surgeon may choose to use skin staples or clips.

Mattress continuous suture

Connected mattress stitches with a knot at the beginning and end

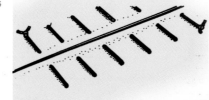

Plain continuous suture

Connected stitches with the thread knotted at the beginning and end of the suture; also called a *continuous running suture*

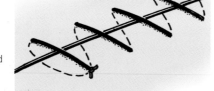

Blanket continuous suture

Looped stitches with a knot at the beginning and end

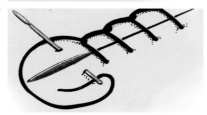

Mattress interrupted suture

Independent stitches with both threads crossing beneath the suture line, leaving only a small portion of suture exposed on each side of the wound

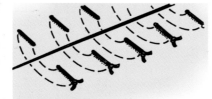

Plain interrupted suture

Individual sutures sewn with a separate piece of thread; half the thread length crosses under the suture line and the other half crosses above the skin surface

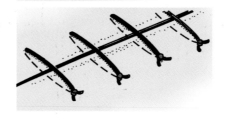

Suture materials

Nonabsorbable sutures

- Used to close the skin surface
- Provide strength and immobility
- Cause minimal tissue irritation
- Consist of silk, cotton, stainless steel, or nylon

Absorbable sutures

- Used when suture removal is undesirable
- Consist of:
  – chromic catgut—a natural catgut treated with chromium trioxide to improve strength and prolong absorption time
  – plain catgut—a material that's absorbed faster and is more likely to cause irritation than chromic catgut
  – synthetic materials (such as polyglycolic acid)—materials that are replacing catgut because they're stronger, more durable, and less irritating.

Caring for and dressing surgical wounds

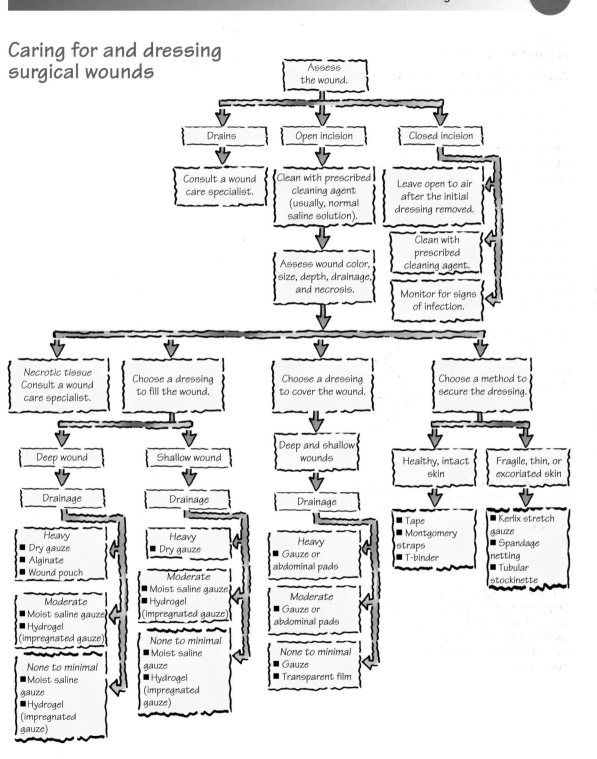

Assess the wound.

Drains
→ Consult a wound care specialist.

Open incision
→ Clean with prescribed cleaning agent (usually, normal saline solution).
→ Assess wound color, size, depth, drainage, and necrosis.

Closed incision
→ Leave open to air after the initial dressing removed.
→ Clean with prescribed cleaning agent.
→ Monitor for signs of infection.

Necrotic tissue Consult a wound care specialist.

Choose a dressing to fill the wound.

Deep wound
→ Drainage
  - Heavy
    - Dry gauze
    - Alginate
    - Wound pouch
  - Moderate
    - Moist saline gauze
    - Hydrogel (impregnated gauze)
  - None to minimal
    - Moist saline gauze
    - Hydrogel (impregnated gauze)

Shallow wound
→ Drainage
  - Heavy
    - Dry gauze
  - Moderate
    - Moist saline gauze
    - Hydrogel (impregnated gauze)
  - None to minimal
    - Moist saline gauze
    - Hydrogel (impregnated gauze)

Choose a dressing to cover the wound.

Deep and shallow wounds
→ Drainage
  - Heavy
    - Gauze or abdominal pads
  - Moderate
    - Gauze or abdominal pads
  - None to minimal
    - Gauze
    - Transparent film

Choose a method to secure the dressing.

Healthy, intact skin
  - Tape
  - Montgomery straps
  - T-binder

Fragile, thin, or excoriated skin
  - Kerlix stretch gauze
  - Spandage netting
  - Tubular stockinette

How to make Montgomery straps

An abdominal dressing requiring frequent changes can be secured with Montgomery straps to promote the patient's comfort. If ready-made straps aren't available, follow these steps to make your own:

1 Cut four to six strips of 2″ to 3″ wide hypoallergenic tape of sufficient length to allow the tape to extend about 6″ (15.2 cm) beyond the wound on each side. (The length of the tape might vary according to the patient's size and the type and amount of dressing.)

2 Fold one of each strip 2″ to 3″ (5 to 7.5 cm) back on itself (sticky sides together) to form a nonadhesive tab. Then cut a small hole in the folded tab's center, close to its top edge. Make as many pairs of straps as you'll need to snugly secure the dressing.

3 Clean the patient's skin to prevent irritation. After his skin dries, apply a skin protectant. Then apply the sticky side of each tape to a skin barrier sheet composed of opaque hydrocolloidal or nonhydrocolloidal materials, and apply the sheet directly to the skin near the dressing.

4 Thread a separate piece of gauze tie, umbilical tape, or twill tape (about 12″ [30.5 cm]) through each pair of holes in the straps, and fasten each tie as you would a shoelace. Don't stress the surrounding skin by securing the ties too tightly.

Replace Montgomery straps every 2 to 3 days or whenever they become soiled. If skin maceration occurs, place new tapes about 1″ (2.5 cm) away from irritation.

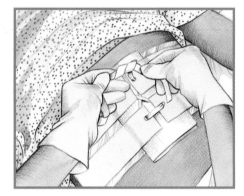

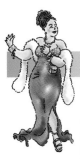

Wound care in bariatric patients

After surgery, bariatric patients experience slower wound healing because:

- Adipose tissue lacks a sufficient blood supply.
- The diaphragm doesn't descend completely, decreasing vital capacity.
- Insufficient oxygen slows digestion of bacteria by neutrophils.

They are also at increased risk for complications, such as:

- trauma (for example, the more forceful retraction needed during surgery may cause necrosis of the abdominal wall)
- infection (the difficulty level of operating on these patients lengthens the operation time, increasing the chances of contamination)
- dehiscence (excess fat and excess blood or serous fluid increase tension on the incision and wound's edges)
- hematoma.

Steps to help prevent complications

- Assess the incision site and vital signs frequently.
- Use an abdominal binder over the surgical site to support the incision.
- Encourage the patient to use deep breathing and spirometry to improve oxygenation.
- Assess nutritional status and promote adequate intake of protein, carbohydrates, and vitamins.

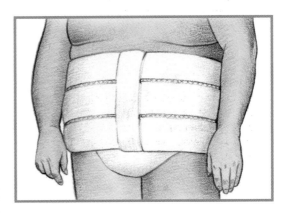

Like a retention wall, retention sutures are used to help "retain" the integrity of a wound.

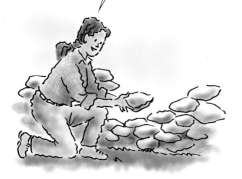

Retention sutures

Although not used exclusively for bariatric patients, retention sutures are sometimes used after surgery in overweight patients to secure a wound's edges and reinforce the suture line. Placed through the abdominal wall before the abdominal layers are closed, they provide support to deep tissue while the more superficial fascia and skin tissue heal.

Surgical drains

Surgeons insert closed-wound drains during surgery when they expect a large amount of postoperative drainage. These drains suction serosanguineous fluid from the wound site.

   If a wound produces heavy drainage, the closed-wound drain may be left in place for longer than 1 week. Drainage must be frequently emptied and measured to maintain maximum suction and prevent strain on the suture line. Treat the tubing exit site as an additional surgical wound.

Purposes

- Promote healing
- Prevent swelling
- Reduce risk of infection and skin breakdown
- Minimize the need for dressing changes

Closed-wound drainage system

A closed-wound drain consists of perforated tubing connected to a portable vacuum unit. (Hemovac and Jackson-Pratt are the most commonly used drainage systems.) The distal end of the tubing lies within the wound and usually leaves the body from a site other than the primary suture line. The drain is usually sutured to the skin. Shown below is a closed-wound drainage system in a postmastectomy patient.

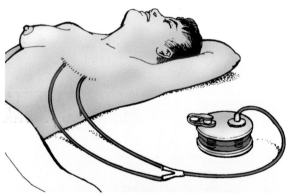

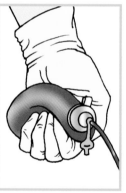

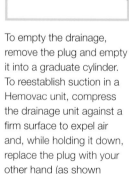

To empty the drainage, remove the plug and empty it into a graduate cylinder. To reestablish suction in a Hemovac unit, compress the drainage unit against a firm surface to expel air and, while holding it down, replace the plug with your other hand (as shown above).

Follow a similar procedure to reestablish suction in a Jackson-Pratt bulb drain (shown above).

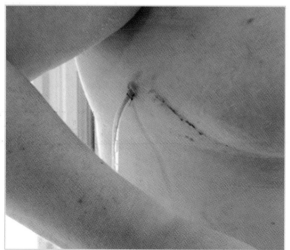

Surgical drain

Colostomy and ileostomy care

A patient with a colostomy or ileostomy wears an external pouch over the ostomy site, attached via a hydrocolloid wafer. The pouch collects fecal matter, helps control odor, and protects the stoma and peristomal skin. Most disposable pouching systems can be used for 7 days, unless a leak develops.

When selecting a pouching system, choose one that delivers the best adhesive seal and skin protection for that patient. Other considerations include the stoma's location and structure, consistency of the fecal matter, availability and cost of supplies, amount of time the patient will wear the pouch, any known adhesive allergy, and the personal preferences of the patient.

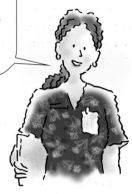

The best time to change a pouching system is first thing in the morning or 2 to 4 hours after meals, when the bowel is least active. After a few months, most patients can predict the time that's best for them.

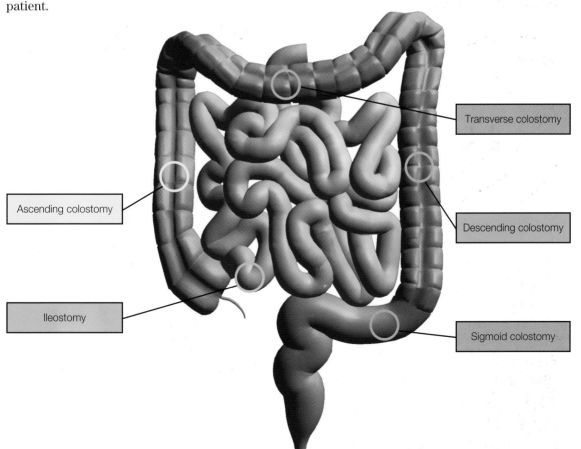

Transverse colostomy

Ascending colostomy

Descending colostomy

Ileostomy

Sigmoid colostomy

Comparing ostomy pouching systems

Manufactured in many shapes and sizes, ostomy pouches are fashioned for comfort, safety, and easy application. Some commonly available pouches are described here.

Disposable pouches

The patient who must empty his pouch often (because of diarrhea or a new colostomy or ileostomy) may prefer a one-piece, drainable, disposable pouch with a closure clamp attached to a skin barrier. This pouch may be used permanently or temporarily, until stoma size stabilizes.

Also disposable and made of transparent or opaque odor-proof plastic, a one-piece disposable closed-end pouch may come with a carbon filter for gas release. A patient with a regular bowel elimination pattern may choose this style for additional security and confidence.

A two-piece disposable drainable pouch with separate skin barrier permits frequent changes and also minimizes skin breakdown.

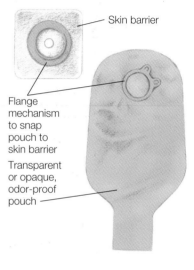

Skin barrier

Flange mechanism to snap pouch to skin barrier

Transparent or opaque, odor-proof pouch

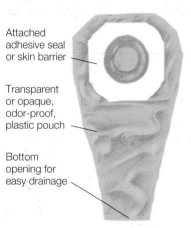

Attached adhesive seal or skin barrier

Transparent or opaque, odor-proof, plastic pouch

Bottom opening for easy drainage

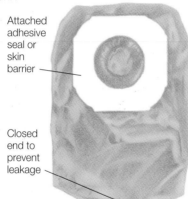

Attached adhesive seal or skin barrier

Closed end to prevent leakage

Reusable pouches

Reusable pouches come with a separate custom-made faceplate and O-ring (as shown at right). Some pouches have a pressure valve for releasing gas. The device has a 1- to 2-month life span, depending on how frequently the patient empties the pouch.

Reusable equipment may benefit a patient who needs a firm faceplate or who wishes to minimize cost. However, many reusable ostomy pouches aren't odor-proof.

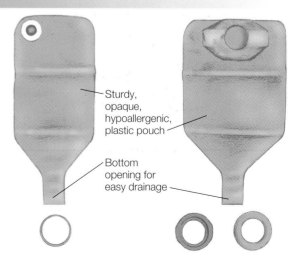

Sturdy, opaque, hypoallergenic, plastic pouch

Bottom opening for easy drainage

Applying a skin barrier and pouch

Fitting a skin barrier and ostomy pouch properly can be done in a few steps. Shown here is a two-piece pouching system with flanges, which is commonly used.

1 Measure the stoma using a measuring guide.

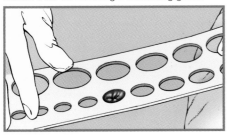

2 Trace the appropriate circle carefully on the back of the skin barrier.

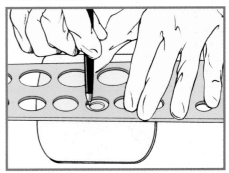

3 Cut the circular opening in the skin barrier. Bevel the edges to keep them from irritating the patient.

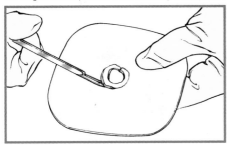

4 Remove the backing from the skin barrier and moisten it or apply barrier paste, as needed, along the edge of the circular opening.

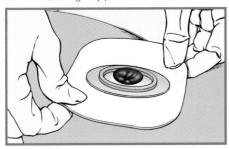

5 Center the skin barrier over the stoma, adhesive side down, and gently press it to the skin.

6 Gently press the pouch opening onto the ring until it snaps into place.

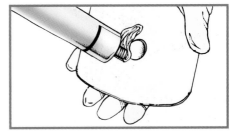

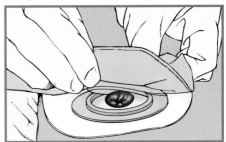

VISION QUEST

Show and tell

Identify the type of burn shown in each of these photos.

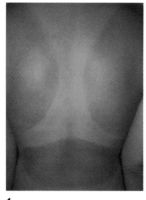

1. _____

_____

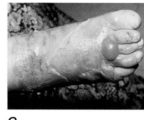

2. _____

_____

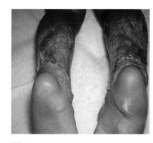

3. _____

_____

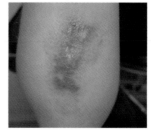

4. _____

_____

Matchmaker

Match the five suture methods shown here with their names.

1.
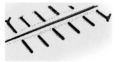
___

2.
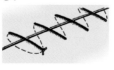
___

3.
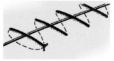
___

4.
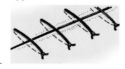
___

5.
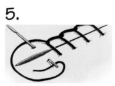
___

A. Mattress interrupted suture
B. Plain interrupted suture
C. Plain continuous suture
D. Mattress continuous suture
E. Blanket continuous suture

Answers: Show and tell 1. First-degree burn, 2. Deep partial-thickness burn, 3. Third-degree burn, 4. Second-degree burn; Matchmaker 1. D, 2. A, 3. C, 4. B, 5. E.

6
Pressure ulcers

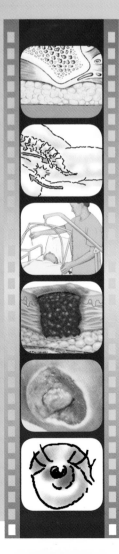

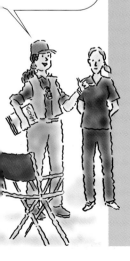

Okay, the pressure is on. In this scene, you'll be caring for patients with pressure ulcers.

Causes

Pressure ulcers typically occur when pressure compresses soft tissue over a bony prominence. Friction and shear also contribute to the development of pressure ulcers.

Understanding the pressure gradient

A V-shaped pressure gradient results from the upward force exerted by a support surface and the downward force of a bony prominence. Pressure is greatest on tissues at the apex of the gradient and lessens to the right and left of this point.

An estimated 1 million to 1.7 million pressure ulcers occur each year in the United States, with one-half of those being stage II or greater.

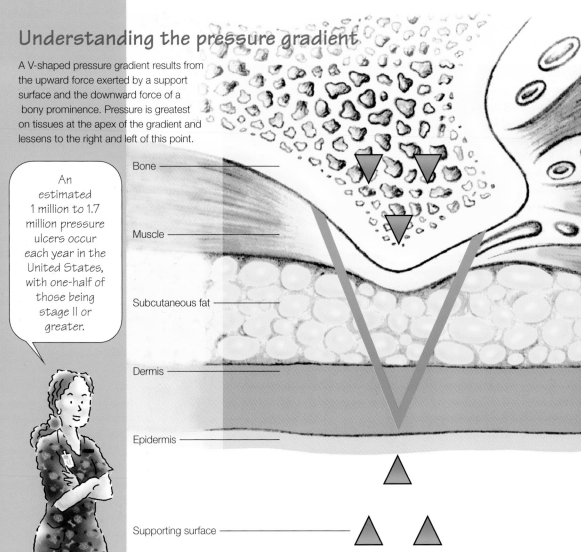

Bone

Muscle

Subcutaneous fat

Dermis

Epidermis

Supporting surface

Sitting

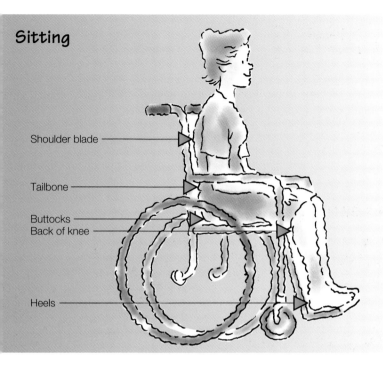

Shoulder blade

Tailbone

Buttocks
Back of knee

Heels

Lying

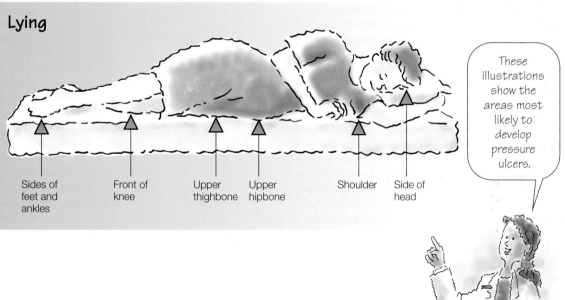

Sides of
feet and
ankles

Front of
knee

Upper
thighbone

Upper
hipbone

Shoulder

Side of
head

These illustrations show the areas most likely to develop pressure ulcers.

Understanding shearing force

Shear is a mechanical force that occurs parallel, rather than perpendicular, to an area of tissue. In this illustration, gravity pulls the body down the incline of the bed. The skeleton and attached tissues move, but the skin remains stationary, held in place by friction between the skin and the bed linen. The skeleton and attached tissues actually slide within the skin, causing the skin to pucker in the gluteal area.

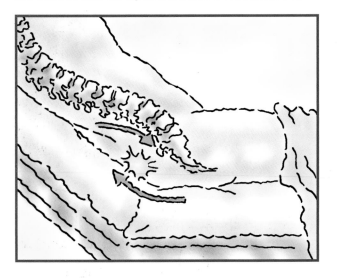

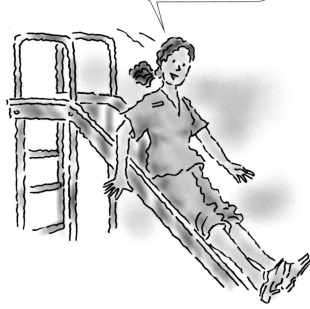

The "Shear" truth is that shearing force causes the skeleton and tissues to slide while the skin remains still.

Risk factors

High-risk patients, whether in an institution or at home, should be assessed regularly for pressure ulcers. Be sure to consider all risk factors when assessing patients.

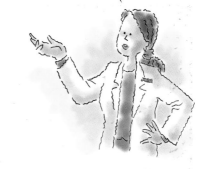

Risk factor	Considerations
Advanced age	▪ Skin becomes more fragile as epidermal turnover slows, vascularization decreases, and skin layers adhere less securely to one another. ▪ Older adults have less lean body mass and less subcutaneous tissue to cushion bony areas. ▪ Underlying problems that increase pressure ulcer risk include poor hydration and impaired respiratory and immune systems.
Immobility	▪ Immobility may be the greatest risk factor for pressure ulcer development. ▪ The patient is less able to move in response to pressure sensations and his position is changed less frequently.
Incontinence	▪ Incontinence increases a patient's exposure to moisture and, over time, increases his risk of skin breakdown. ▪ Urinary and fecal incontinence can result in excessive moisture and chemical irritation (fecal incontinence can cause more damage because of pathogens in stools).
Infection	▪ Compressed skin has a lower local resistance to bacterial infection. ▪ Infection may reduce the pressure needed to cause tissue necrosis.
Low blood pressure	▪ Low blood pressure can lead to tissue ischemia, particularly in patients with vascular disorders. ▪ As tissue perfusion drops, the skin is less tolerant of sustained external pressure, increasing the risk of damage from ischemia.
Malnutrition	▪ A strong correlation exists between poor nutrition and the development of pressure ulcers. ▪ The body requires increased protein for healing; malnutrition can lead to decreased protein levels, including decreased albumin. ▪ A direct correlation exists between pressure ulcer stage and the degree of hypoalbuminemia.

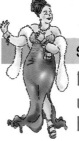

Special attention

Pressure ulcers in bariatric patients

Bariatric patients are at increased risk for pressure ulcer development for several reasons:

■ Their nutritional status might not be optimum.

■ They're prone to developing protein malnutrition during metabolic stress (even though they may have excess body fat storage).

■ Adipose tissue commonly has decreased vascularity.

■ They're unable to change position or move independently due to immobility.

■ The moist environment in skinfolds promotes bacterial growth, which can lead to fungal infections and decreased skin integrity.

Braden Scale for Predicting Pressure Sore Risk

Tally the numbers for each description that applies to your patient. Determine your patient's risk as follows:

- 15 to 18: At risk
- 13 to 14: Moderate risk
- 10 to 12: High risk
- 9 or below: Very high risk.

Sensory perception: Ability to respond meaningfully to pressure-related discomfort

1. Completely limited	2. Very limited
Unresponsive (does not moan, flinch, or grasp) to painful stimuli due to diminished level of consciousness or sedation OR Limited ability to feel pain over most of body	Responds only to painful stimuli. Cannot communicate discomfort except by moaning or restlessness. OR Has a sensory impairment which limits the ability to feel pain or discomfort over $1/2$ of body.

Moisture: Degree to which skin is exposed to moisture

1. Constantly moist	2. Very moist
Skin is kept moist almost constantly by perspiration, urine, etc. Dampness is detected every time patient is moved or turned.	Skin is often, but not always moist. Linen must be changed at least once a shift.

Activity: Degree of physical activity

1. Bedfast	2. Chairfast
Confined to bed.	Ability to walk severely limited or nonexistent. Cannot bear own weight and/or must be assisted into chair or wheelchair.

Mobility: Ability to change and control body position

1. Completely immobile	2. Very limited
Does not make even slight changes in body or extremity position without assistance.	Makes occasional slight changes in body or extremity position but unable to make frequent or significant changes independently.

Nutrition: <u>Usual</u> food intake pattern

1. Very poor	2. Probably inadequate
Never eats a complete meal. Rarely eats more than $1/3$ of any food offered. Eats 2 servings or less of protein (meat or dairy products) per day. Takes fluids poorly. Does not take a liquid dietary supplement. OR Is NPO and/or maintained on clear liquids or IVs for more than 5 days.	Rarely eats a complete meal and generally eats only about $1/2$ of any food offered. Protein intake includes only 3 servings of meat or dairy products per day. Occasionally will take a dietary supplement. OR Receives less than optimum amount of liquid diet or tube feeding.

Friction and shear

1. Problem	2. Potential problem
Requires moderate to maximum assistance in moving. Complete lifting without sliding against sheets is impossible. Frequently slides down in bed or chair, requiring frequent repositioning with maximum assistance. Spasticity, contractures, or agitation leads to almost constant friction.	Moves feebly or requires minimum assistance. During a move skin probably slides to some extent against sheets, chair, restraints or other devices. Maintains relatively good position in chair or bed most of the time but occasionally slides down.

Copyright 1988. Barbara Braden and Nancy Bergstrom. Reprinted with permission. All rights reserved.
Permission to use this tool in clinical practice may be obtained, usually free of charge, at www.bradenscale.com.

Patient's name _____ Evaluator's name _____

	Date of assessment		

3. Slightly limited
Responds to verbal commands but cannot always communicate discomfort or the need to be turned.
OR
Has some sensory impairment which limits ability to feel pain or discomfort in 1 or 2 extremities.

4. No impairment
Responds to verbal commands. Has no sensory deficit which would limit ability to feel or voice pain or discomfort.

3. Occasionally moist
Skin is occasionally moist, requiring an extra linen change approximately once a day.

4. Rarely moist
Skin is usually dry; linen only requires changing only at routine intervals.

3. Walks occasionally
Walks occasionally during day, but for very short distances, with or without assistance. Spends majority of each shift in a bed or chair.

4. Walks frequently
Walks outside room at least twice a day and inside room at least once every two hours during waking hours.

3. Slightly limited
Makes frequent though slight changes in body or extremity position independently.

4. No limitations
Makes major and frequent changes in position without assistance.

> The Braden scale is the most widely used scale in the United States for determining a patient's risk of pressure ulcers.

3. Adequate
Eats over half of most meals. Eats a total of 4 servings of protein (meat, dairy products) per day. Occasionally will refuse a meal, but will usually take a supplement when offered.
OR
Is on a tube feeding or TPN regimen which probably meets most of nutritional needs.

4. Excellent
Eats most of every meal. Never refuses a meal. Usually eats a total of 4 or more servings of meat and dairy products. Occasionally eats between meals. Does not require supplementation.

3. No apparent problem
Moves in bed and in chair independently and has sufficient muscle strength to lift up completely during move. Maintains good position in bed or chair.

Total score

Norton scale

Total the numbers from each category that describes your patient. A score of 14 or less indicates a risk of developing pressure ulcers.

Physical condition		Mental condition		Activity		Mobility		Incontinence		
Good	4	Alert	4	Ambulatory	4	Full	4	None	4	
Fair	3	Apathetic	3	Walk/help	3	Slightly limited	3	Occasional	3	**Total score**
Poor	2	Confused	2	Chairbound	2	Very limited	2	Usually-urine	2	
Very bad	1	Stuporous	1	Bedridden	1	Immobile	1	Urine/feces	1	

Name:　　　　　Date:

Name:　　　　　Date:

Name:　　　　　Date:

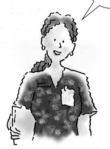

> The Norton scale is another scale recommended to determine a patient's risk of pressure ulcers.

When to assess and reassess

How frequently you assess and reassess your patient for pressure ulcer risk will depend on the care setting. The Agency for Healthcare Research and Quality and the Wound, Ostomy, and Continence Nurses Society recommend the following intervals:

■ *Acute care:* Upon admission and then every 24 to 48 hours or when the patient's condition changes

■ *Long-term care:* Upon admission and then weekly for the first 4 weeks and monthly to quarterly after that; also whenever the patient's condition changes

■ *Home health care:* Upon admission and at every visit.

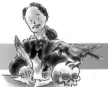

take note

Pressure ulcer documentation

5/6/11	1415	Nursing admit note: Received pt. from ED at 1300. Sacral pressure ulcer noted: 5½ cm length, 3 cm width, 0.4 cm depth. Tunneling present between 9 and 10 o'clock, measuring 2 cm in depth. Small amount of serosanguineous drainage oozing from wound bed. No odor present. Ulcer bed is red with granulation tissue. Thin band (approximately 0.5 cm) of yellow slough present around entire ulcer margin. Surrounding skin pink and intact, except for 1-cm area of induration at 4 o'clock. Pt. reported ulcer pain as 7 on 0-to-10 scale. Hydrocodone administered at 1330 per order. Pt. now reports pain as 3 on 0-to-10 scale. Wound/ostomy nurse N. Cooper paged to evaluate pt. and determine wound care plan. Wet-to-moist dressing applied and pt. positioned off of ulcer until evaluation. *L. Bradley, RN*

Prevention

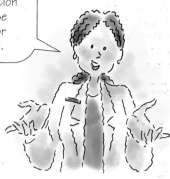

Preventing pressure ulcers—which includes identifying patients at risk and taking action to minimize those risks—is a major health care goal.

Managing the intensity and duration of pressure is key to preventing pressure ulcers, especially for patients with limited mobility. Other prevention strategies include reducing friction and shear, minimizing moisture, maximizing nutritional status, and controlling chronic illnesses that contribute to pressure ulcer development (such as diabetes).

Positioning patients

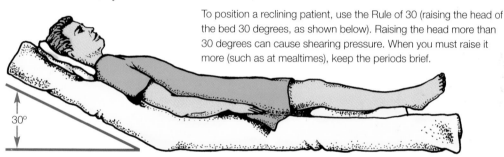

To position a reclining patient, use the Rule of 30 (raising the head of the bed 30 degrees, as shown below). Raising the head more than 30 degrees can cause shearing pressure. When you must raise it more (such as at mealtimes), keep the periods brief.

30°

When repositioning a patient from the left side to the right, make sure his weight rests on the buttock, not the hipbone. This reduces pressure on the trochanter and sacrum. The angle between the bed and an imaginary lateral line through the hips should be about 30 degrees (as shown here).

If needed, use pillows or a foam wedge to help the patient maintain the proper position. Cushion pressure points, such as the knees and shoulders, with pillows.

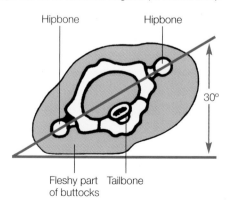

Hipbone   Hipbone

30°

Fleshy part   Tailbone
of buttocks

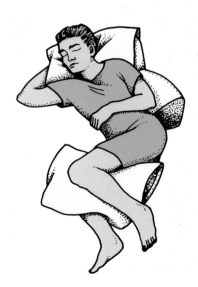

Pressure ulcer prevention algorithm

| Provide patient teaching. | ← **Yes** | Risk for activity or mobility deficit? | **No** → | Reassess periodically. |

Yes

Assess pressure ulcer risk using an assessment tool.

| Incontinence or moisture problems? | Sensory perception, mobility, and activity deficits? | Nutritional deficits? |

No / **Yes** — **Yes** / **No** — **Yes** / **No**

| Reassess periodically. | Clean skin immediately when soiled. | Elevate the head of the bed no more than 30 degrees. | Reassess periodically. | Consult a nutritionist for a nutritional assessment. | Reassess periodically. |

| Use a commercial moisture barrier. | Use preventive devices, such as a turn sheet or mechanical lift device. | Increase protein intake and increase calorie intake, if needed. |

| Use absorbent pads or diapers that hold moisture. | Pad bony prominences and keep the patient's heels off the bed. | Maintain adequate hydration. |

| Offer a bedpan or urinal at regular intervals. | Develop a turning schedule based on the patient's needs. |

Consult a wound care specialist for appropriate pressure-relieving devices and surfaces and for further assessment.

Consult a physical therapist to help increase mobility.

Comparing support surface characteristics

Characteristics	Support devices					
	Air-fluidized bed	Low-air-loss bed	Alternating air mattress	Static flotation (air or water)	Foam overlay mattress	Standard mattress
Increased support area	✔	✔	✔	✔	✔	✘
Low moisture retention	✔	✔	✘	✘	✘	✘
Reduced heat accumulation	✔	✔	✘	✘	✘	✘
Shear reduction	✔	??	✔	✔	✘	✘
Pressure redistribution	✔	✔	✔	✔	✔	✘
Dynamic	✔	✔	✔	✘	✘	✘
Cost per day	$$$$$	$$$$$	$$$	$	$	$

Air-fluidized therapy bed

The fluidlike surface of an air-fluidized therapy bed redistributes pressure on the skin, thereby helping prevent pressure ulcers and promote wound healing. The bed also provides the advantages of flotation without the disadvantages of instability, patient positioning difficulties, and immobility.

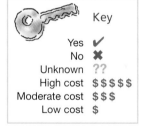

Key

Yes	✔
No	✘
Unknown	??
High cost	$$$$$
Moderate cost	$$$
Low cost	$

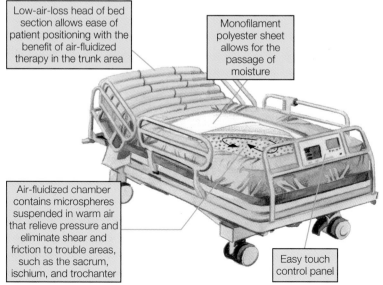

Low-air-loss head of bed section allows ease of patient positioning with the benefit of air-fluidized therapy in the trunk area

Monofilament polyester sheet allows for the passage of moisture

Air-fluidized chamber contains microspheres suspended in warm air that relieve pressure and eliminate shear and friction to trouble areas, such as the sacrum, ischium, and trochanter

Easy touch control panel

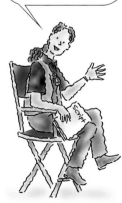

Just as actors need emotional support to combat psychological pressure, patients need physical support to combat pressure ulcers.

Low-air-loss therapy bed

Low-air-loss therapy beds contain segmented air cushions that inflate to help redistribute pressure on skin surfaces and to minimize shearing force during repositioning. The beds also circulate cool air to promote evaporation and temperature reduction, which helps prevent maceration. These mattresses fit on regular hospital bed frames.

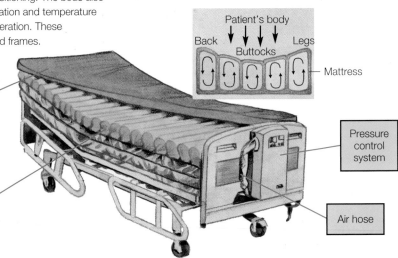

Patient's body
Back   Buttocks   Legs
Mattress

Air- and vapor-permeable, water-resistant fabric covering helps reduce friction and shear

Air circulates through these cushions and conforms to the patient's body, evenly distributing pressure

Pressure control system

Air hose

Alternating pressure mattress

An alternating pressure mattress contains chambers filled with air or water that periodically circulates to create alternating low- and high-pressure areas. This action redistributes pressure while stimulating blood circulation.

Some alternating pressure mattress models also include low-air-loss therapy.

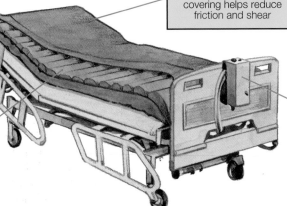

Air- and vapor-permeable, water-resistant fabric covering helps reduce friction and shear

Electric pump circulates air or water

Chambers filled with air or water alternately inflate and deflate to create high- and low-pressure areas

Using a hydraulic lift

Using a hydraulic lift to transfer an immobile or obese patient reduces the effects of shear and friction on the skin—a key strategy of pressure ulcer prevention. These general guidelines will help you to transfer your patient safely and comfortably. Be sure to follow the manufacturer's instructions.

After placing the patient in a supine position in the center of the sling, position the hydraulic lift above him (as shown below). Then attach the chains to the hooks on the sling.

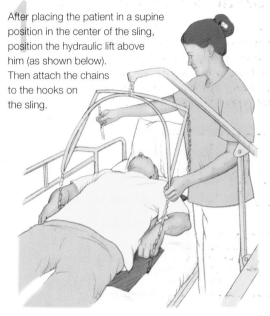

Turn the lift handle clockwise to raise the patient to the sitting position. If he's positioned properly, continue to raise him until he's suspended just above the bed.

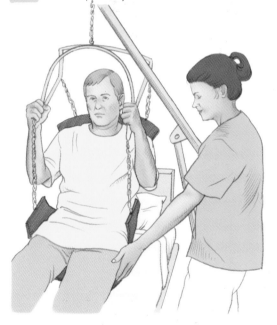

After positioning the patient above the wheelchair, turn the lift handle counterclockwise to lower him onto the seat. When the chains become slack, stop turning and unhook the sling from the lift.

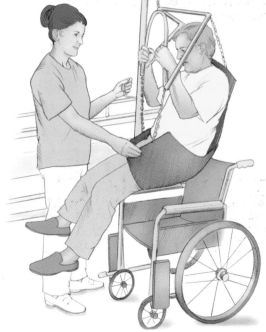

Assessment

The Pressure Ulcer Scale for Healing (PUSH) tool can help you monitor, reassess, and document pressure ulcers.

Assess pressure ulcers weekly. A well-vascularized pressure ulcer without infection should show signs of healing within 2 weeks. If not, reevaluate the care plan.

PUSH tool

Patient's name: _____   Patient ID #: _____

Ulcer location: _____   Date: _____

Directions

Observe and measure the pressure ulcer. Categorize the ulcer with respect to surface area, exudate, and type of wound tissue. Record a subscore for each of the ulcer characteristics. Add the subscores to obtain the total score. A comparison of total scores measured over time provides an indication of the improvement or deterioration in pressure ulcer healing.

Length × width

0 cm^2	1 < 0.3 cm^2	2 0.3 to 0.6 cm^2	3 0.7 to 1 cm^2	4 1.1 to 2 cm^2	5 2.1 to 3 cm^2
	6 3.1 to 4 cm^2	7 4.1 to 8 cm^2	8 8.1 to 12 cm^2	9 12.1 to 24 cm^2	10 > 24 cm^2

Subscore [ ]

Exudate amount

0 None	1 Light	2 Moderate	3 Heavy	—	—

Subscore [ ]

Tissue type

0 Closed	1 Epithelial tissue	2 Granulation tissue	3 Slough	4 Necrotic tissue	—

Subscore [ ]

Total score [ ]

Length × width

Measure the greatest length (head-to-toe) and the greatest width (side-to-side) using a centimeter ruler. Multiply these two measurements (length × width) to obtain an estimate of surface area in square centimeters (cm^2). Don't guess! Always use a centimeter ruler and always use the same method each time you measure.

Exudate amount

Estimate the amount of exudate (drainage) present after removing the dressing and before applying any topical agent to the ulcer. Estimate as none, light, moderate, or heavy.

Tissue type

This refers to the types of tissue in the wound bed. Score as a 4 if you note necrotic tissue. Score as a 3 if you observe slough but no necrotic tissue. Score a clean wound that contains granulation tissue as a 2. Score a superficial wound that's reepithelializing as a 1. When the wound is closed, score it as a 0. The following guide describes each tissue type:

4—Necrotic tissue (eschar): Black, brown, or tan tissue that adheres firmly to the wound bed or ulcer edges and may be either firmer or softer than surrounding tissue

3—Slough: Yellow or white tissue that adheres to the ulcer bed in strings or thick clumps or is mucinous

2—Granulation tissue: Pink or beefy red tissue with a shiny, moist, granular appearance

1—Epithelial tissue: For superficial ulcers, new pink or shiny tissue (skin) that grows in from the edges or as islands on the ulcer surface

0—Closed or resurfaced: Completely covered wound with epithelium (new skin).

Staging

Pressure ulcer staging reflects the depth and extent of tissue involvement. The classification system developed by the National Pressure Ulcer Advisory Panel (NPUAP) is the most widely used system for staging pressure ulcers. The NPUAP recently redefined its pressure ulcer stages by adding two new stages for deep tissue injury and unstageable ulcers.

Suspected deep tissue injury

Deep tissue injury is characterized by a purple or maroon localized area of intact skin or blood-filled blister caused by damage of underlying soft tissue from pressure or shear. The injury may be preceded by tissue that's painful, firm, mushy, boggy, or warm or cool compared to adjacent tissue. As the wound evolves, it may become a thin blister over a dark wound bed or become covered by a thin layer of eschar. Even with optimal treatment, rapid exposure of additional layers of tissue can occur. Deep tissue injury may be difficult to detect in individuals with dark skin tones.

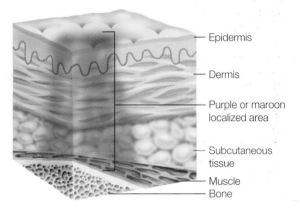

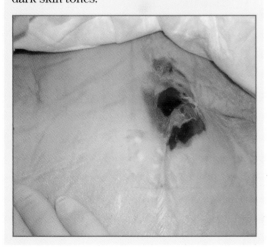

Stage I

Stage I ulcers are characterized by intact skin with nonblanchable redness of a localized area, usually over a bony prominence. Darkly pigmented skin may not have visible blanching, but its color may differ from the surrounding area.

To identify a stage I pressure ulcer, compare the suspected area to an adjacent area or to the same region on the other side of the body. Indications of a stage I pressure ulcer include differences in:
- skin temperature (warmth or coolness)
- tissue consistency (firm)
- sensation (pain).

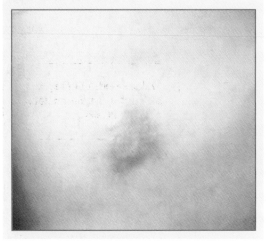

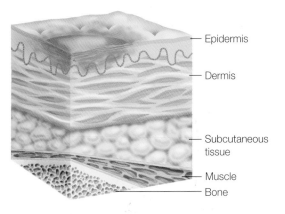

Stage II

A stage II pressure ulcer is characterized by partial-thickness loss of the dermis, presenting as a shallow, open ulcer with a red-pink wound bed without slough. It may also present as an intact or open serum-filled blister.

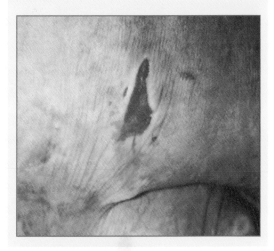

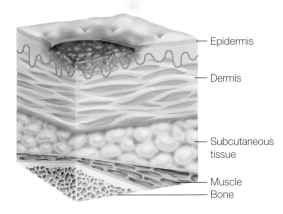

Stage III

A stage III pressure ulcer is characterized by full-thickness tissue loss. Subcutaneous fat may be visible, but bone, tendon, and muscle aren't exposed. Slough may be present but doesn't obscure the depth of tissue loss. Undermining and tunneling may be present. The depth of a stage III ulcer varies by anatomical location.

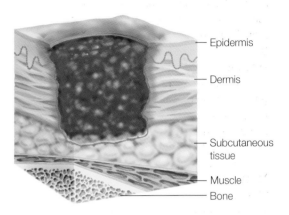

Epidermis

Dermis

Subcutaneous tissue

Muscle

Bone

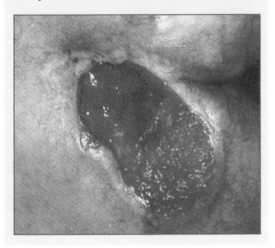

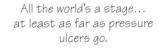

All the world's a stage... at least as far as pressure ulcers go.

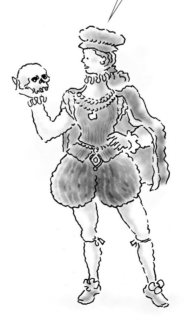

Stage IV

A stage IV pressure ulcer involves full-thickness tissue loss with exposed bone, tendon, or muscle. Slough or eschar may be present on some parts of the wound bed. Undermining and tunneling are also common. The depth of a stage IV ulcer varies by anatomical location.

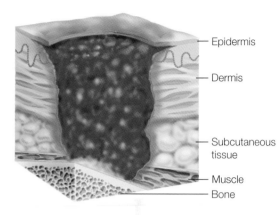

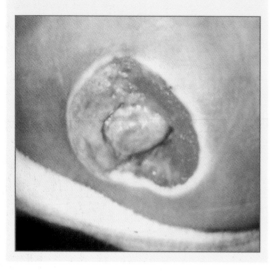

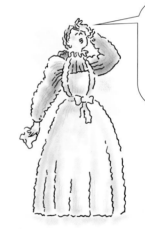

Alas, some pressure ulcers are unstageable until slough and eschar are removed.

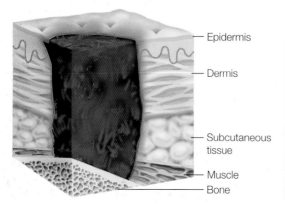

Unstageable

An unstageable ulcer is characterized by full-thickness tissue loss in which the base of the ulcer in the wound bed is covered by slough (yellow, tan, gray, green, or brown), eschar (tan, brown, or black), or both. Until enough slough or eschar is removed to expose the base of the wound, the true depth, and therefore stage, can't be determined.

Treatment

Treatment of pressure ulcers includes nutritional assessment and support, management of tissue loads, ulcer care, and management of bacterial colonization and infection.

Management of pressure ulcers algorithm

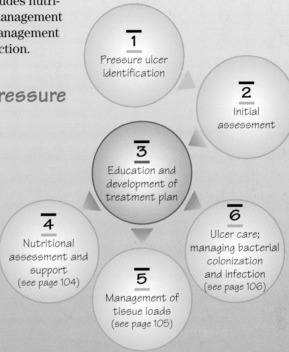

1. Pressure ulcer identification

2. Initial assessment

3. Education and development of treatment plan

4. Nutritional assessment and support (see page 104)

5. Management of tissue loads (see page 105)

6. Ulcer care; managing bacterial colonization and infection (see page 106)

7. Is ulcer healing?

Yes

No

8. Monitor

9. Reassessment of treatment plan and evaluation of adherence

Return to 3

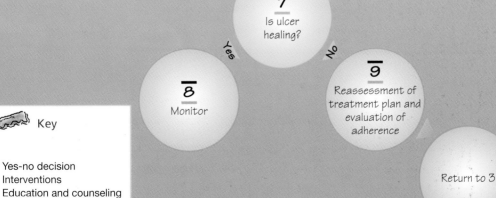

Key

Yes-no decision
Interventions
Education and counseling
Refer to previous node

Nutritional assessment and support algorithm

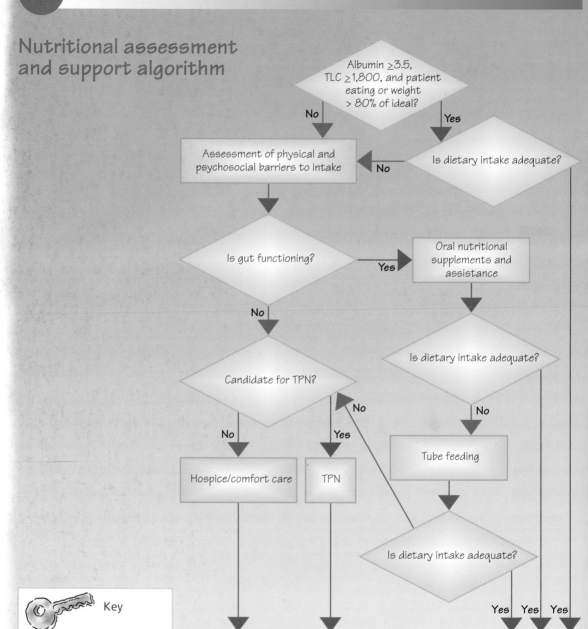

Key

Yes-no decision
Interventions

Note:
TLC = Total lymphocyte count
TPN = Total parenteral nutrition

Management of tissue loads algorithm

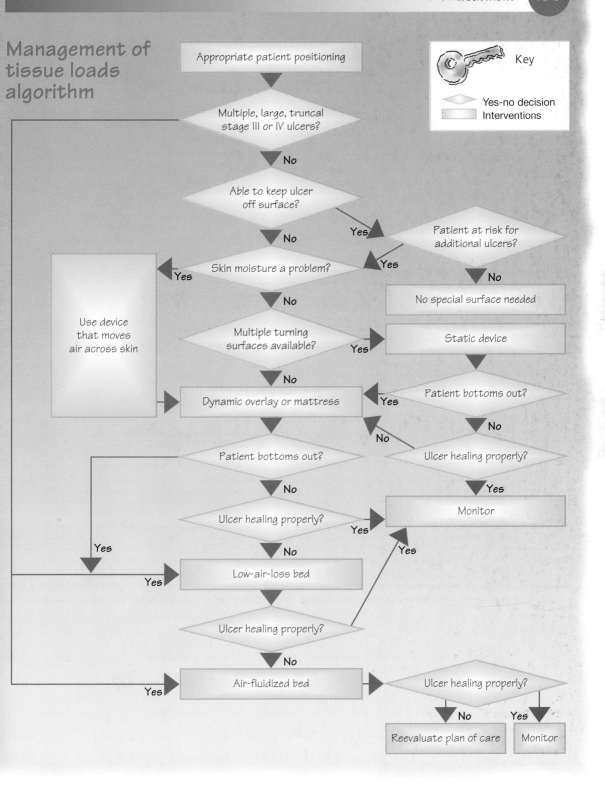

Key
◇ Yes-no decision
▭ Interventions

Appropriate patient positioning

Multiple, large, truncal stage III or IV ulcers? → No

Able to keep ulcer off surface? → Yes → Patient at risk for additional ulcers? → Yes / No → No special surface needed

Able to keep ulcer off surface? → No

Skin moisture a problem? → Yes → Use device that moves air across skin

Skin moisture a problem? → No

Multiple turning surfaces available? → Yes → Static device → Patient bottoms out? → Yes → Dynamic overlay or mattress / No → Ulcer healing properly? → Yes → Monitor / No

Multiple turning surfaces available? → No → Dynamic overlay or mattress

Patient bottoms out? → Yes / No

Patient bottoms out? → No → Ulcer healing properly? → Yes → Monitor / No → Low-air-loss bed

Ulcer healing properly? → No → Low-air-loss bed → Ulcer healing properly? → Yes → Monitor / No → Air-fluidized bed

Air-fluidized bed → Ulcer healing properly? → No → Reevaluate plan of care / Yes → Monitor

Managment of bacterial colonization and infection algorithm

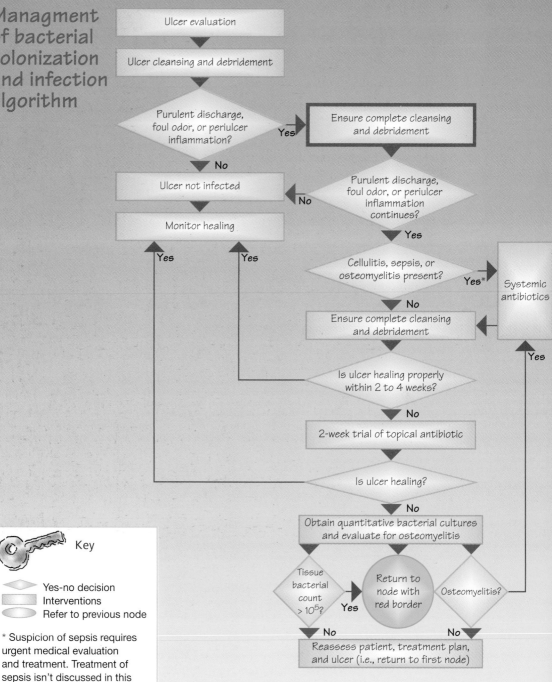

Ulcer evaluation

Ulcer cleansing and debridement

Purulent discharge, foul odor, or periulcer inflammation?

Yes → Ensure complete cleansing and debridement

No

Ulcer not infected

Monitor healing

Purulent discharge, foul odor, or periulcer inflammation continues?

No

Yes

Cellulitis, sepsis, or osteomyelitis present?

Yes* → Systemic antibiotics

No

Ensure complete cleansing and debridement

Is ulcer healing properly within 2 to 4 weeks?

Yes

No

2-week trial of topical antibiotic

Is ulcer healing?

Yes

No

Obtain quantitative bacterial cultures and evaluate for osteomyelitis

Tissue bacterial count > 10^5?

Yes → Return to node with red border

Osteomyelitis?

Yes

No

No

Reassess patient, treatment plan, and ulcer (i.e., return to first node)

Key

◇ Yes-no decision
▭ Interventions
⬭ Refer to previous node

* Suspicion of sepsis requires urgent medical evaluation and treatment. Treatment of sepsis isn't discussed in this guideline.

Pressure ulcer care

Assess for signs of pressure injury.

Stage I	Stage II, stage III, or stage IV

Wash with soap and warm water; dry thoroughly.	Irrigate wound bed with normal saline solution or ordered solution. Wash around wound bed with normal saline solution; dry thoroughly.

Remove area from pressure sources.

Assess other contributing factors to break in skin integrity.

Remediate other factors, if possible.

Assess color, odor, and amount of drainage on old dressing.

Assess ulcer color, length, width, depth, and drainage.

Assess for necrotic areas.

Choose method of debridement (surgical or nonsurgical).

Assist with surgical debridement if ordered.

Assess skin around wound. (Is it intact, macerated, inflamed, tunneled?)

Choose care for periwound skin. (Keep dry, use protective barrier, avoid adhesives?)

Choose type of ulcer treatment. (Add moisture, remove moisture, use antibacterial, fill cavity, support autolysis of debris, totally occlude, partially occlude?)

Choose a dressing. (Primary with separate secondary, combination?) Initiate and maintain pressure preventive measures and remediation of any other contributing factors, if possible.

Regularly reassess effectiveness of interventions.

VISION QUEST

Matchmaker

Match the four illustrations of pressure ulcers with their correct stage.

1. 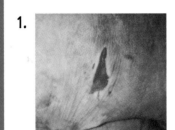 ___

2. 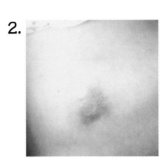 ___

3. 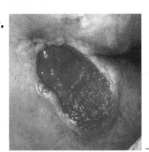 ___

4. 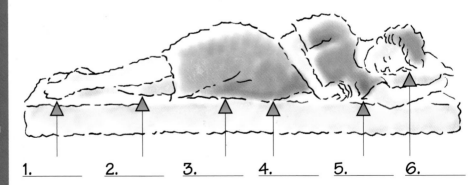 ___

A. Stage I
B. Stage II
C. Stage III
D. Stage IV

Able to label?

Label the pressure points susceptible to ulcer formation in the illustration.

1. _____ 2. _____ 3. _____ 4. _____ 5. _____ 6. _____

Answers: Matchmaker 1. B, 2. A, 3. D, 4. C; Able to label? 1. Sides of feet and ankles, 2. Front of knee, 3. Upper thighbone, 4. Upper hipbone, 5. Shoulder, 6. Side of head.

7
Vascular ulcers

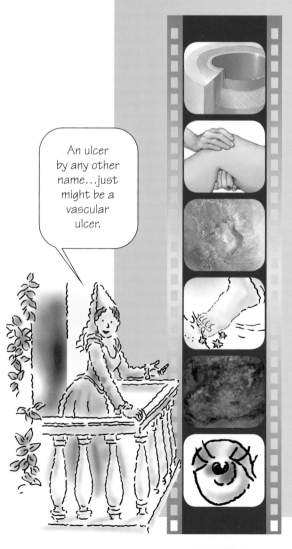

An ulcer by any other name...just might be a vascular ulcer.

Vascular system

The body's vascular system consists of:
- veins (carry blood toward the heart)
- arteries (carry blood away from the heart)
- lymphatic system (a separate circulatory system that collects waste products and delivers them to the venous system).

Veins

Veins carry deoxygenated blood back to the heart for reoxygenation.

A close look at a vein

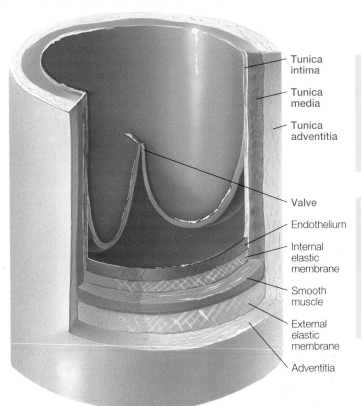

Tunica intima

Tunica media

Tunica adventitia

Valve

Endothelium

Internal elastic membrane

Smooth muscle

External elastic membrane

Adventitia

Vein walls have three layers. Compared to arteries of the same size, veins have thinner walls and wider diameters.

Veins have a unique system of cup-shaped valves that open toward the heart. The valves function to keep blood flowing in one direction—toward the heart.

Major lower limb veins

Venous ulcers most commonly occur in the lower extremities. The illustration below shows the major veins in this part of the body.

Types of veins

The lower portion of the body contains three major types of veins.

Superficial veins

Superficial veins lie just beneath the skin; they drain through perforator veins into deep veins.

Perforator veins

Perforator veins connect superficial to deep veins.

Deep veins

Deep veins receive venous blood from perforator veins and return it to the heart.

He's really a superficial vein. He just thinks if he reads enough literature, people will start to think he's deep.

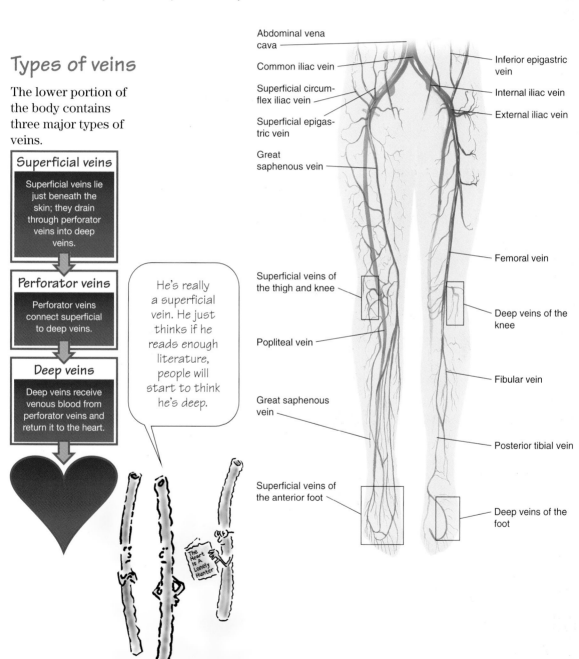

- Abdominal vena cava
- Common iliac vein
- Superficial circumflex iliac vein
- Superficial epigastric vein
- Great saphenous vein
- Inferior epigastric vein
- Internal iliac vein
- External iliac vein
- Femoral vein
- Superficial veins of the thigh and knee
- Deep veins of the knee
- Popliteal vein
- Fibular vein
- Great saphenous vein
- Posterior tibial vein
- Superficial veins of the anterior foot
- Deep veins of the foot

Arteries

Arteries carry blood from the heart to every functioning cell in the body. The lower portion of the body receives its arterial flow through the abdominal aorta and the major arteries branching from it.

A close look at an artery

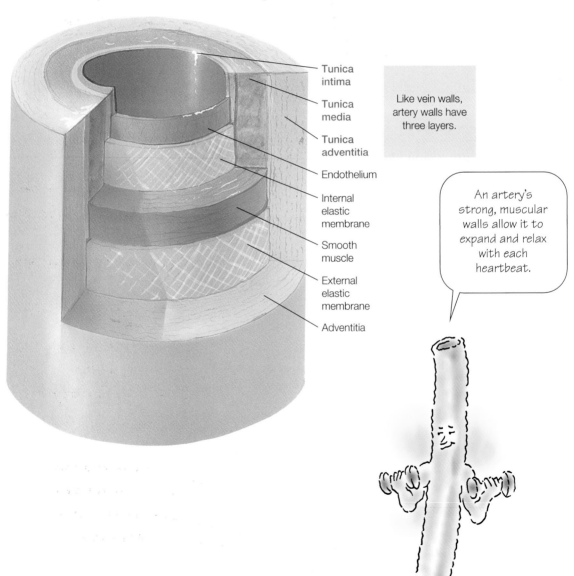

Tunica intima

Tunica media

Tunica adventitia

Endothelium

Internal elastic membrane

Smooth muscle

External elastic membrane

Adventitia

Like vein walls, artery walls have three layers.

An artery's strong, muscular walls allow it to expand and relax with each heartbeat.

Major lower limb arteries

Arterial ulcers most commonly occur in the lower extremities. This illustration identifies the major arteries in the lower portion of the body.

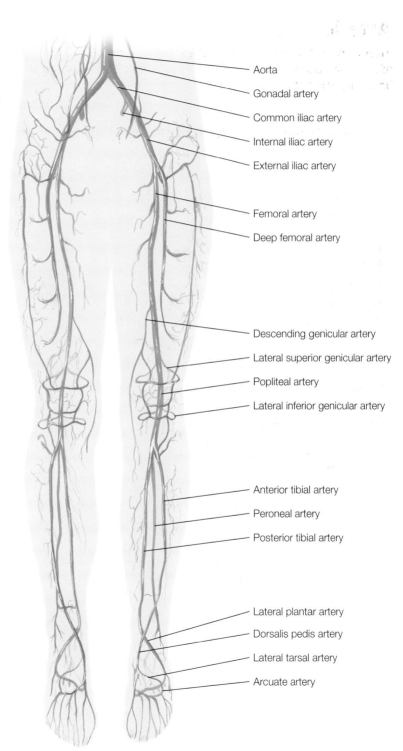

- Aorta
- Gonadal artery
- Common iliac artery
- Internal iliac artery
- External iliac artery
- Femoral artery
- Deep femoral artery
- Descending genicular artery
- Lateral superior genicular artery
- Popliteal artery
- Lateral inferior genicular artery
- Anterior tibial artery
- Peroneal artery
- Posterior tibial artery
- Lateral plantar artery
- Dorsalis pedis artery
- Lateral tarsal artery
- Arcuate artery

Assessing lower extremity pulses

Assessing pulses is an effective way to evaluate arterial blood flow to the lower extremities. These illustrations show where to position your fingers when palpating for pulses of the lower extremities. Use your index and middle fingers to apply pressure.

Femoral pulse

Press relatively hard at a point inferior to the inguinal ligament. For obese patients, palpate in the groin crease, halfway between the pubic bone and hip bone.

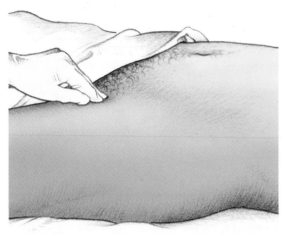

Popliteal pulse

Press firmly in the popliteal fossa at the back of the knee.

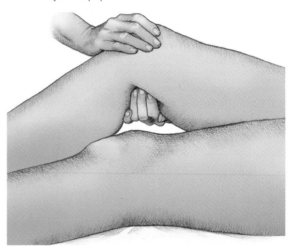

Dorsalis pedis pulse

Place your fingers on the medial dorsum of the foot while the patient points his toes down. The pulse is difficult to palpate here and may seem absent in healthy patients.

Posterior tibial pulse

Apply pressure behind and slightly below the medial malleolus.

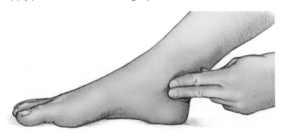

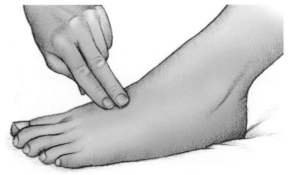

Lymphatic system

The lymphatic system is a vascular network that drains lymph (a protein-rich fluid similar to plasma) from body tissues and intravascular compartments and returns it to the venous system.

Lymphatic system and drainage route

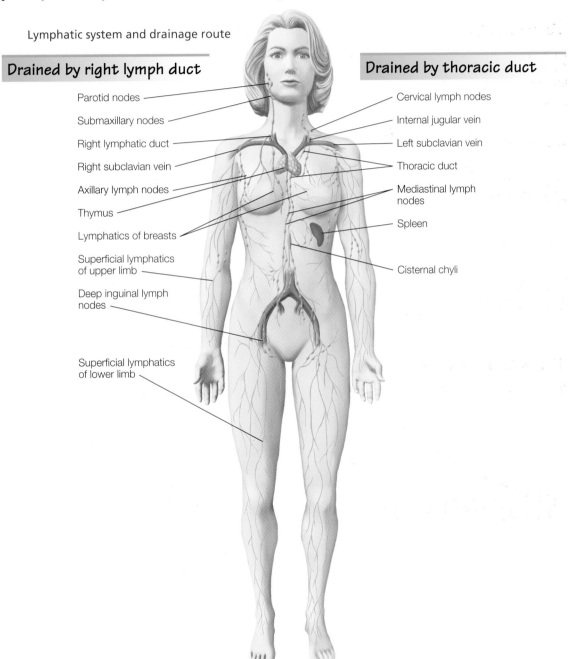

Drained by right lymph duct

- Parotid nodes
- Submaxillary nodes
- Right lymphatic duct
- Right subclavian vein
- Axillary lymph nodes
- Thymus
- Lymphatics of breasts
- Superficial lymphatics of upper limb
- Deep inguinal lymph nodes
- Superficial lymphatics of lower limb

Drained by thoracic duct

- Cervical lymph nodes
- Internal jugular vein
- Left subclavian vein
- Thoracic duct
- Mediastinal lymph nodes
- Spleen
- Cisternal chyli

The lymphatic system begins peripherally, with lymph capillaries that absorb fluid. The capillaries proceed centrally to thin vascular vessels. These vessels empty into collecting ducts, which empty into major veins at the base of the neck.

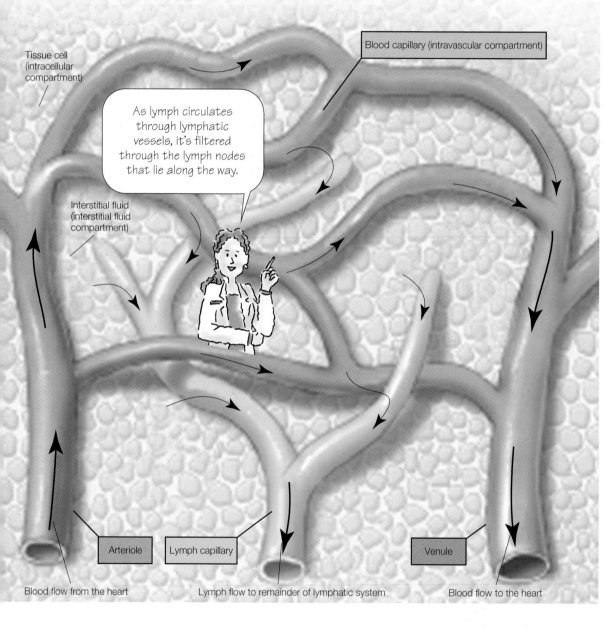

Using a Doppler to assess blood flow

In Doppler ultrasonography, high-frequency sound waves are used to assess blood flow. A handheld transducer, or probe, directs the sound waves into a vessel, where they strike moving red blood cells (RBCs). The frequency of the sound waves changes in proportion to the velocity of the RBCs. Doppler ultrasonography can be used to assess both arterial and venous blood flow.

Assessing arterial blood flow

- Apply a small amount of transmission gel to the ultrasound probe.
- Position the probe on the skin directly over the selected artery.
- Turn the instrument on and set the volume to the lowest setting.
- To obtain the best signal, tilt the probe at a 45-degree angle from the artery, making sure that the gel is between the skin and the probe.
- Slowly move the probe in a circular motion to locate the center of the artery.
- Listen for a triphasic, biphasic, or monophasic sound, which occurs when the Doppler signal isolates an artery.
- Count the signal for 60 seconds to determine the pulse rate.

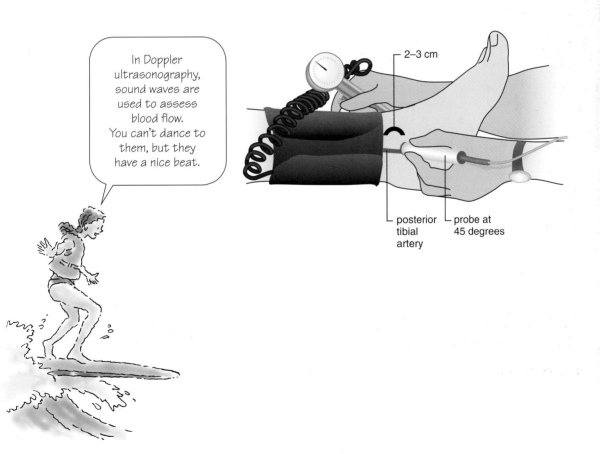

In Doppler ultrasonography, sound waves are used to assess blood flow. You can't dance to them, but they have a nice beat.

2–3 cm

posterior tibial artery

probe at 45 degrees

Measuring ankle-brachial index

The ankle-brachial index (ABI) is a value derived from blood pressure measurements that shows the progress or improvement of arterial disease. Each value in the index is a ratio of blood pressure measurement in the affected limb to the highest systolic pressure in the brachial arteries.

Steps

- Place the patient in a supine position with the legs at heart level.
- Measure and record both brachial blood pressures.
- Wrap the blood pressure cuff around one ankle, just above the malleolus, with the cuff bladder centered over the posterior tibial artery.
- Apply ultrasound transmission gel to a Doppler transducer.
- Hold the Doppler transducer over the dorsalis pedis or posterior tibial artery at a 45-degree angle.
- Inflate the blood pressure cuff until the Doppler signal disappears.
- Slowly deflate the cuff until the Doppler signal returns.
- Record the pressure as the ankle systolic pressure.
- Repeat the process using the dorsalis pedis artery.
- Calculate the ABI by dividing the highest ankle pressure by the highest brachial systolic pressure.
- Repeat the process on the contralateral limb.

Interpretation of results

- ABI > 0.9 = Normal
- ABI 0.71 to 0.9 = Mild arterial insufficiency
- ABI 0.41 to 0.7 = Moderate arterial insufficiency
- ABI 0 to 0.40 = Severe arterial insufficiency

The ABI may not be accurate in patients with diabetes or arterial medial calcinosis.

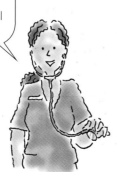

Ankle-brachial index (ABI) worksheet

Patient Name _____

Date _____   Patient number _____

Right Arm
Systolic Pressure:
_____

Left Arm
Systolic Pressure:
_____

Right Ankle
Systolic Pressure:

Left Ankle
Systolic Pressure:

Posterior tibial (PT) ———
Dorsal pedis (DP) ———

——— Posterior tibial (PT)
——— Dorsal pedis (DP)

Right ABI
$$\frac{\text{Higher Right Ankle Pressure}}{\text{Higher Arm Pressure}} = \frac{\text{mm Hg}}{\text{mm Hg}} = \underline{\quad}$$

Left ABI
$$\frac{\text{Higher Right Ankle Pressure}}{\text{Higher Arm Pressure}} = \frac{\text{mm Hg}}{\text{mm Hg}} = \underline{\quad}$$

Example
$$\frac{\text{Higher Ankle Pressure}}{\text{Higher Brachial Pressure}} \quad \frac{\text{mm Hg}}{\text{mm Hg}} \quad \underline{\quad}$$

Vascular ulcers

Disorders of the venous, arterial, and lymphatic systems can cause chronic wounds, called *vascular ulcers*, to develop.

> Venous and arterial ulcers tend to occur on the distal portion of the legs, whereas lymphatic ulcers occur on either the arms or the legs.

Types of vascular ulcers

Type of ulcer	Typical location	Clinical findings
Venous	■ Anywhere from ankle to midcalf ■ Most common on medial aspect of ankle above the malleolus	■ Irregular shape ■ Dry, crusted or moist, slightly macerated borders ■ Shallow wound base covered with beefy red granulation tissue, yellow film, or gray necrotic tissue (black necrotic tissue rarely present except in acute injury) ■ Edema (one of the first signs of venous disease) ■ Hyperpigmentation in calves due to buildup of hemosiderin (results from breakdown of red blood cells that have leaked into tissue) ■ Atrophie blanche (spots of ivory white plaque in skin, usually surrounded by hyperpigmentation) ■ Dull, aching pain or heaviness that is relieved by elevation of the leg
Arterial	■ Tips of toes, corners of nail beds on toes, over bony prominences, and between toes	■ Pale or mottled wound ■ Well-demarcated wound edges ■ Dry wound base with no granulation tissue (due to impaired blood flow to tissue) ■ Presence of necrotic tissue (commonly) ■ Surrounding skin that feels cooler than normal on palpation ■ Dependent rubor (ischemic skin becomes deep red when patient places his foot in a dependent position) ■ Thin, pale yellow nails (may be thickened as a result of fungal infection) ■ History of claudication (pain distal to a narrowed artery brought on by exercise and relieved by rest) and rest pain (commonly occurs in foot when patient is asleep; alleviated by lowering extremity)
Lymphatic	■ Arms and legs, most commonly ankle area	■ Shallow ulcer bed that may be oozing, moist, or blistered ■ Firm, fibrotic surrounding skin that's thickened by edema ■ Cellulitis (possibly)

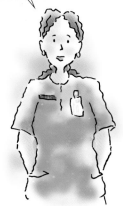

Between 70% and 90% of all leg ulcers are venous ulcers.

Venous ulcers

When leg veins fail to propel a sufficient supply of blood back to the heart, blood begins to pool in the legs (venous insufficiency). Causes of venous insufficiency include:

■ **incompetent valves**—most common cause; can result when a blood clot disrupts valve function or when a vein distends (venous hypertension) to the point that the valve no longer closes completely

■ **inadequate calf muscle function.**

Signs of venous insufficiency

Physical activity is crucial to adequate venous return. Leg muscle paralysis or prolonged inactivity can drastically hinder the amount of blood returning to the heart.

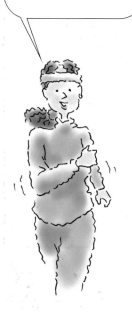

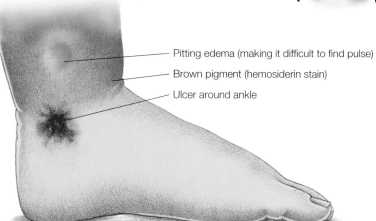

Pitting edema (making it difficult to find pulse)

Brown pigment (hemosiderin stain)

Ulcer around ankle

Other signs and symptoms of venous insufficiency

■ Fibrotic skin
A buildup of fibrin causes skin and subcutaneous tissue to thicken and become fibrotic—a condition called *lipodermatosclerosis.* The skin eventually develops a shiny, taut appearance.

■ Eczema
Eczema (venous dermatitis) commonly occurs, particularly in patients with recurrent ulcers. Skin over scar tissue and edematous tissue is fragile. Drainage from larger ulcers—or medications themselves—can irritate the skin and aggravate eczema.

■ Telangiectasia
The superficial veins just below the skin's surface become dilated, producing a weblike appearance on the skin.

■ Hemosiderosis
A brown discoloration of the skin occurs just above the ankle as a result of hemosiderin deposits.

A closer look at venous ulcers

Venous ulcers most commonly occur above the medial malleolus. These ulcers have irregular borders and typically appear moist.

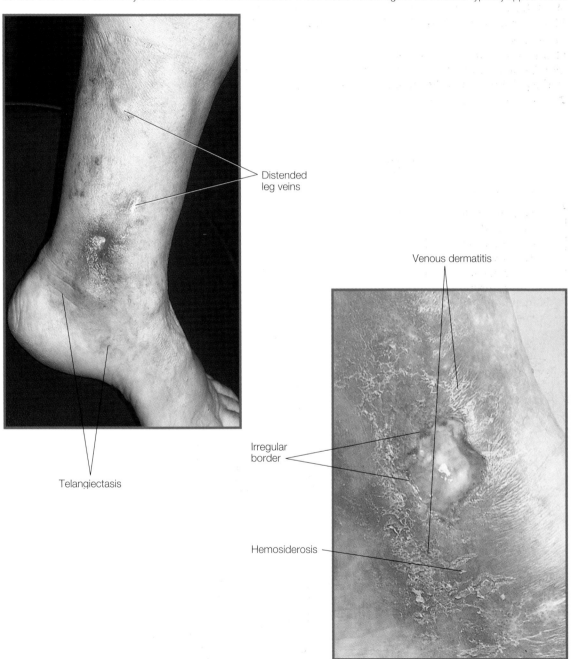

Distended
leg veins

Telangiectasis

Venous dermatitis

Irregular
border

Hemosiderosis

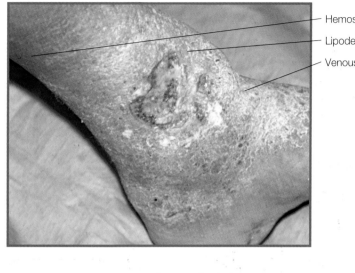

Hemosiderosis

Lipodermatosclerosis

Venous dermatitis

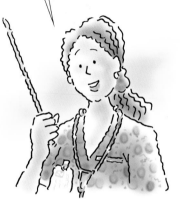

Note the common characteristics of venous ulcers in these photographs: moist, beefy red wound base; hemosiderosis; and lipodermatosclerosis.

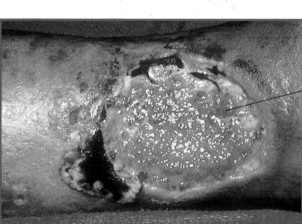

Moist, beefy red wound base

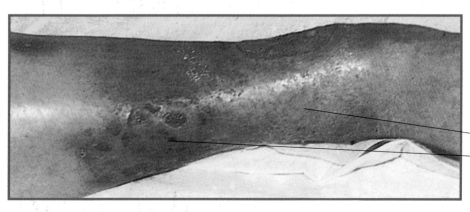

Lipodermatosclerosis

Hemosiderosis

Arterial ulcers

Also called *ischemic ulcers*, arterial ulcers result from tissue ischemia caused by insufficient blood flow through an artery (arterial insufficiency). Causes of arterial insufficiency include arterial stenosis (narrowing) or obstruction (from thrombosis, emboli, atherosclerosis, vasculitis, or Raynaud's phenomenon). Arterial ulcers most commonly occur in the area around the toes.

Development of an arterial ulcer

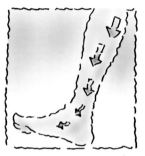

Arterial flow is diminished.

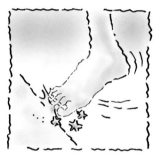

Trauma occurs to an area with arterial insufficiency.

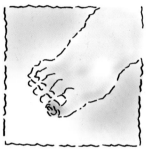

Reduced blood flow impairs healing, and a chronic wound results.

The most common cause of arterial ulcers is atherosclerosis, so stay back, plaque.

Understanding atherosclerosis

In atherosclerosis, fatty, fibrous plaques progressively narrow the arterial lumen. This reduces blood flow and leads to tissue ischemia. The illustrations below show the progression of atherosclerosis.

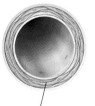

Normal artery

Fatty streak

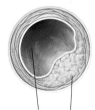

Reduced blood flow

Fibrous plaque

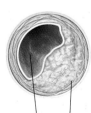

Severely restricted blood flow

Fibrous plaque

Risk factors for atherosclerosis

- Advanced age
- Smoking
- Obesity
- Hyperlipidemia
- Diabetes mellitus
- Hypertension
- Sedentary lifestyle

Signs of arterial insufficiency

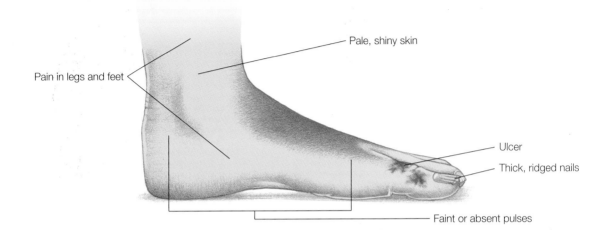

Pale, shiny skin

Pain in legs and feet

Ulcer

Thick, ridged nails

Faint or absent pulses

Identifying dependent rubor

Dependent rubor is a sign of chronic arterial insufficiency. To elicit this sign during a physical examination:

■ Elevate the foot with the ulcer to a 30-degree angle. If the foot is ischemic, the skin will pale.
■ Ask the patient to lower the foot into a dependent position. Ischemic skin becomes deep red as the tissue fills with blood. This dramatic color change—called *dependent rubor*—signifies severe tissue ischemia.

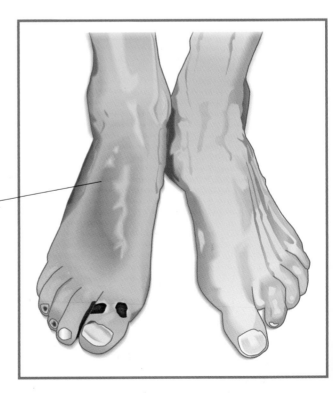

Rubor

A closer look at arterial ulcers

Arterial ulcers have well-demarcated edges. Because of decreased blood flow, the base of the ulcer is typically pale and dry and granulation tissue may be absent. On examination, you may notice an area of wet necrosis or a dry scab. The skin surrounding the ulcer will feel cooler than normal.

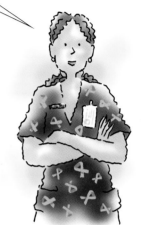

Common sites of arterial ulcers include the tips of the toes, the corners of nail beds on the toes, over bony prominences, and between toes.

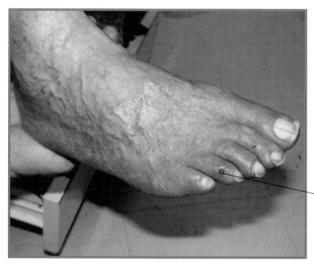

Arterial toe ulcer

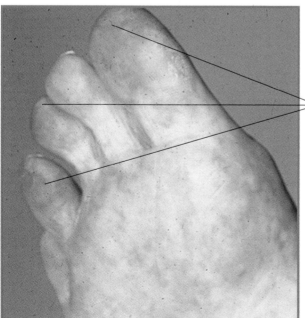

Ulcers resulting from arterial emboli

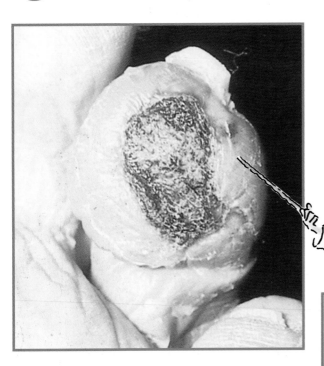

Note the dry, necrotic wound bed on this distal toe ulcer.

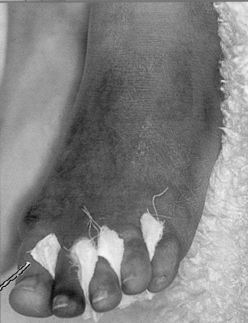

These toes are showing signs of gangrene as a result of severe arterial ischemia.

Lymphatic ulcers

Lymphatic ulcers result when a part of the body afflicted with lymphedema suffers an injury. Here are some predisposing factors for ulcer formation:

■ **Pressure on capillaries**—The skin and underlying tissue in areas with lymphedema become firm and fibrotic over time. This thickened tissue presses on capillaries, occluding blood flow and leaving the area vulnerable to ulcer formation. Because of the poor circulation, these ulcers are extremely difficult to treat.

■ **Skin folds from massive swelling**—Skin folds can trap moisture, leading to tissue maceration and ulcer formation.

■ **Traumatic injury or pressure**—Pressure or injury in an area with lymphedema commonly leads to an ulcer.

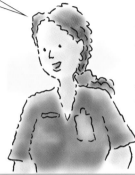

Lymphatic ulcers commonly occur in the ankle area, but they can develop at any site of traumatic injury in an area with lymphedema.

Understanding lymphedema

Lymphedema occurs when an obstruction in the lymphatic system causes lymphatic fluid to build up in the interstitial spaces of body tissues. In the legs, the steady seepage of fluid into interstitial tissues can result in massive edema, as shown here.

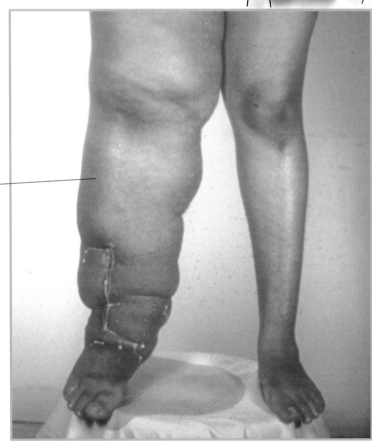

Edema

Signs of lymphedema

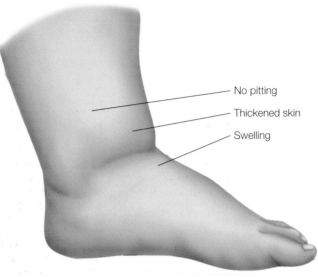

No pitting

Thickened skin

Swelling

A closer look at lymphatic ulcers

Lymphatic ulcers are typically shallow and may be oozing, moist, or blistered. The surrounding skin is usually firm, fibrotic, and thickened by edema. Cellulitis (tissue inflammation) may also be present. Dry, warty spots called *papillomatoses* may develop.

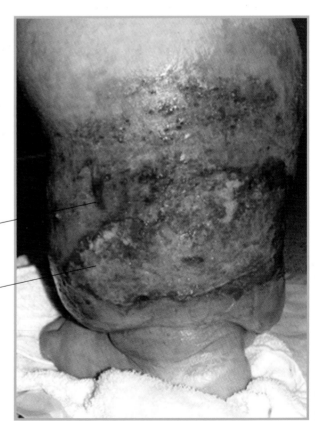

Papillomatosis

Shallow, moist lymphatic ulcer

Treatment

Effective treatment of a vascular ulcer involves caring for the wound as well as managing the underlying vascular disease. The goals and treatment recommendations vary depending on the type of ulcer.

Type of ulcer	Treatment goals	Therapies and procedures	Wound care
Venous	• Control edema • Manage underlying venous disease • Provide appropriate wound care	• Limb elevation to allow gravity to drain fluid from the limb • Compression bandages, layered compression bandages, elastic bandages, compression pumps, compression stockings, or graduated compression support hosiery to reduce edema • Unna's boot to provide compression, protection, and a moist environment for healing	• Apply occlusive dressings to promote moist wound healing, growth of granulation tissue, and reepithelialization. • Apply growth factors to the wound bed, as ordered, to improve healing rate. • Consider application of Apligraf (a bioengineered skin equivalent) for a venous ulcer that fails to heal within 4 weeks of treatment.
Arterial	• Reestablish arterial flow • Provide appropriate wound care	• Arterial bypass to restore arterial flow • Angioplasty (with possible stent insertion) to treat arterial stenosis	• Keep the wound dry and protected from pressure. • As ordered, apply an antiseptic or antimicrobial agent and then place small gauze pads between the toes. Change the pads daily to keep toe ulcers dry. • Never soak arterial ulcers. • If revascularization succeeds, change the type of dressing to keep moist tissue moist and dry tissue dry.
Lymphatic	• Reduce edema • Prevent infection • Provide appropriate wound care	• Limb elevation and compression pump therapy to reduce edema • Comprehensive decongestive therapy (a form of massage) to reduce edema and improve circulation	• Follow guidelines for venous ulcer care. • Choose dressings that can manage large fluid loads while protecting the surrounding skin, such as foams and other absorbent dressings.

Treatment of venous ulcers algorithm

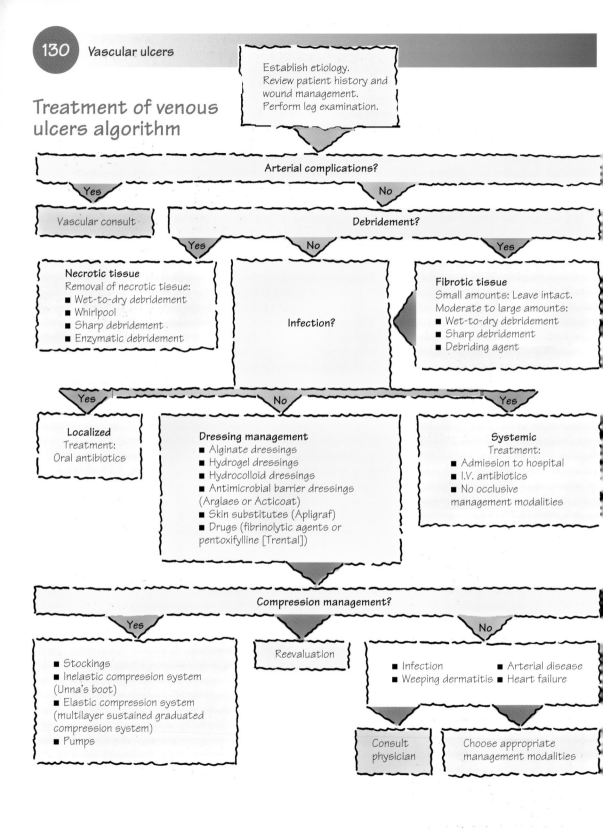

Establish etiology.
Review patient history and
wound management.
Perform leg examination.

Arterial complications?

Yes

No

Vascular consult

Debridement?

Yes

No

Yes

Necrotic tissue
Removal of necrotic tissue:
- Wet-to-dry debridement
- Whirlpool
- Sharp debridement
- Enzymatic debridement

Infection?

Fibrotic tissue
Small amounts: Leave intact.
Moderate to large amounts:
- Wet-to-dry debridement
- Sharp debridement
- Debriding agent

Yes

No

Yes

Localized
Treatment:
Oral antibiotics

Dressing management
- Alginate dressings
- Hydrogel dressings
- Hydrocolloid dressings
- Antimicrobial barrier dressings
(Arglaes or Acticoat)
- Skin substitutes (Apligraf)
- Drugs (fibrinolytic agents or
pentoxifylline [Trental])

Systemic
Treatment:
- Admission to hospital
- I.V. antibiotics
- No occlusive
management modalities

Compression management?

Yes

No

- Stockings
- Inelastic compression system
(Unna's boot)
- Elastic compression system
(multilayer sustained graduated
compression system)
- Pumps

Reevaluation

- Infection
- Weeping dermatitis
- Arterial disease
- Heart failure

Consult
physician

Choose appropriate
management modalities

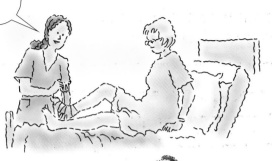

A treatment for venous ulcers involves applying an inelastic compression system called Unna's boot.

How to wrap Unna's boot

- Clean the patient's skin thoroughly.
- Flex the patient's knee.
- With the foot positioned at a right angle to the leg, wrap the medicated gauze bandage firmly—not tightly—around the patient's foot. Make sure the dressing covers the heel.
- Continue wrapping upward, overlapping the layers by 50% with each turn. Make sure the dressing circles the leg at an angle to avoid compromising the circulation. Smooth the boot with your free hand as you go, as shown below.

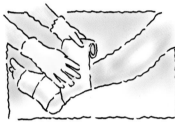

- Stop wrapping about 1" (2.5 cm) below the knee, as shown below. If constriction develops as the dressing hardens, make a 2" (5.1-cm) slit in the boot just below the knee.

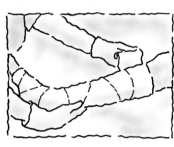

- If drainage is excessive, wrap a roller gauze dressing over the boot.
- Finally, wrap the boot with an elastic bandage in a figure-eight pattern, as shown below.

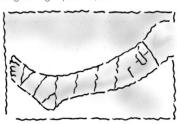

take note

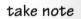

Documenting Unna's boot application

1/2/11	1030	Unna's boot applied to pt's right leg at 0930. Ulcer above right medial malleolus measures 3 cm length, 1.5 cm width, 0.2 cm depth. Wound bed appears moist and beefy red. No drainage or odor noted. Surrounding skin dry and scaly but intact. Right lower extremity pulses easily palpable. Wound cleaned with NSS and allowed to dry thoroughly. Medicated gauze bandage applied on right leg from just above the toes to the knee, then covered with elastic bandage. Assisted patient in elevation of right leg to allow for drying. Toes on right foot presently appear pink with immediate capillary refill, no edema, normal sensation. Pt. tolerated procedure well. ———— Isa Rapp, R.N.

Treatment of arterial ulcers algorithm

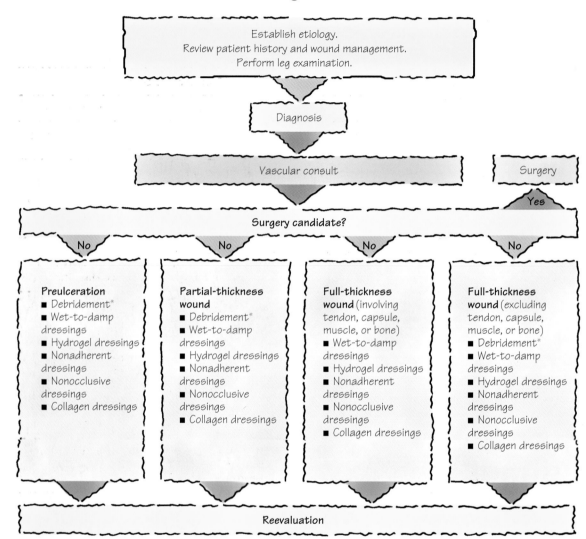

Establish etiology.
Review patient history and wound management.
Perform leg examination.

Diagnosis

Vascular consult

Surgery

Yes

Surgery candidate?

No

No

No

No

Preulceration
- Debridement*
- Wet-to-damp dressings
- Hydrogel dressings
- Nonadherent dressings
- Nonocclusive dressings
- Collagen dressings

Partial-thickness wound
- Debridement*
- Wet-to-damp dressings
- Hydrogel dressings
- Nonadherent dressings
- Nonocclusive dressings
- Collagen dressings

Full-thickness wound (involving tendon, capsule, muscle, or bone)
- Wet-to-damp dressings
- Hydrogel dressings
- Nonadherent dressings
- Nonocclusive dressings
- Collagen dressings

Full-thickness wound (excluding tendon, capsule, muscle, or bone)
- Debridement*
- Wet-to-damp dressings
- Hydrogel dressings
- Nonadherent dressings
- Nonocclusive dressings
- Collagen dressings

Reevaluation

* Debride only arterial ulcers with necrotic tissue. Be careful not to disturb the already compromised arteries.

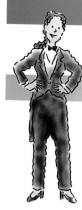

Best dressed

Dressings for vascular ulcers

Dressing	Indications and contraindications		
	VENOUS ULCERS	ARTERIAL ULCERS	LYMPHATIC ULCERS
Alginate	▪ Use to manage copious drainage.	▪ Use isn't indicated.	▪ Use for heavily draining wounds.
Foam	▪ Use to protect the ulcer. ▪ Use for absorption underneath a compression dressing.	▪ Use to protect the ulcer. ▪ Use with dry gangrene. ▪ Use for a moist, revascularized ulcer.	▪ Use to protect the ulcer. ▪ Use to absorb drainage.
Gauze	▪ Use for absorption.	▪ Use for protection and to allow dry gangrene to maintain its dryness.	▪ Use for absorption or padding (don't allow it to dry out on the ulcer).
Hydrocolloid	▪ Use to promote granulation. ▪ Use to manage pain. ▪ Don't use when copious drainage is present.	▪ Use for autolytic debridement. ▪ Use for primary dressing after revascularization. ▪ Don't use on ischemic tissue. ▪ Don't use when infection or cellulitis is present.	▪ Use to protect the skin. ▪ Use to promote epithelialization. ▪ Don't use when copious drainage is present. ▪ Don't use when cellulitis is present.
Hydrogel	▪ Don't use when copious drainage is present.	▪ Use to maintain a moist wound bed. ▪ Use to debride.	▪ Use to manage pain. ▪ Use to debride.
Transparent film	▪ Use isn't indicated.	▪ Use only after the ulcer has almost completely healed.	▪ Use to protect fragile skin.

VISION QUEST

Matchmaker

Match the three types of ulcers shown here with their names.

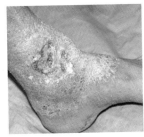 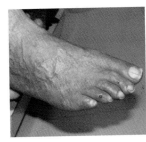 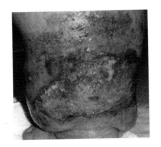

1. _____

2. _____

3. _____

A. Arterial ulcer
B. Lymphatic ulcer
C. Venous ulcer

My word!

Use the clues to help you unscramble the names of the major cause of each type of vascular ulcer. Then use the circled letters to answer the question posed.

Question: **What is the most common type of vascular ulcer?**

1. **What disorder is the major cause of arterial ulcers?**

cherriesalossto

_ _ _ _ _ _ _ _ _ _ _ _ ◯ _ _ ◯

2. **What disorder is the major cause of venous ulcers?**

conceiveiffunnyisus

◯ _ _ ◯ _   _ ◯ _ _ _ _ _ _ _ _

3. **What disorder is the major cause of lymphatic ulcers?**

playmedhem

_ _ _ _ _ ◯ _ _ _ _

Answers: Matchmaker 1. C, 2. A, 3. B; My word! 1. Atherosclerosis, 2. Venous insufficiency, 3. Lymphedema; Question: Venous.

8
Diabetic foot ulcers

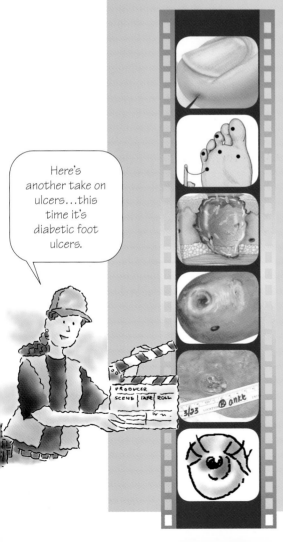

Here's another take on ulcers...this time it's diabetic foot ulcers.

Causes

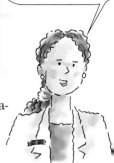

About 23 million adults and children in the United States have diabetes. Of those, 15% will develop diabetic foot ulcers.

Diabetes mellitus—a metabolic disorder characterized by hyperglycemia—occurs because of a lack of insulin, a lack of insulin effect, or both. The high plasma glucose levels resulting from diabetes commonly damage blood vessels and nerves, leading to poor circulation and decreased sensation. This typically occurs in the lower extremities, leaving patients with diabetes at risk for developing foot ulcers.

Understanding diabetic trineuropathy

Uncontrolled diabetes commonly results in three concurrent neuropathies that dramatically increase a patient's risk of developing diabetic foot ulcers.

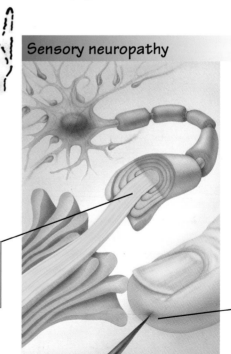

Sensory neuropathy

Ischemia or demyelination causes nerve death or deterioration…

…which results in decreased pain sensation.

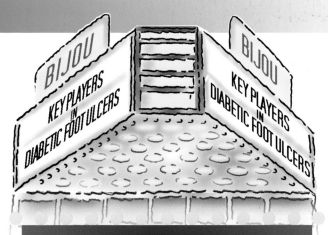

■ **Diabetic neuropathy:** a nerve disorder causing impaired or lost function in tissue served by affected nerve fibers
■ **Pressure, friction, and shear:** pressure and mechanical forces that can lead to foot ulcers in patients with neuropathy
■ **Peripheral vascular disease:** disorder that impairs healing of existing ulcers and can also contribute to neuropathy

Motor neuropathy

Muscular atrophy in the plantar surface of the foot results in increased arch height and clawed toes.

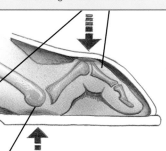

In addition, the fat pad that normally covers the metatarsal heads migrates toward the toes, exposing the heads to pressure and increasing ulcer risk.

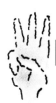

Autonomic neuropathy

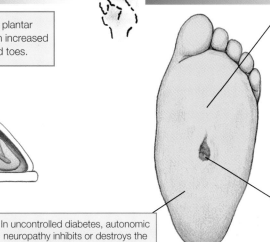

In Charcot's disease, bones weakened by osteopenia suffer fractures that the patient doesn't feel because of sensory neuropathy. Over time, this process causes bony dissolution that culminates with the collapse of the midfoot into a rocker bottom deformity.

In uncontrolled diabetes, autonomic neuropathy inhibits or destroys the sympathetic component of the autonomic nervous system, which controls vasoconstriction in peripheral blood vessels. The resulting unfettered flow of blood to the lower limbs and feet may cause osteopenia in foot and ankle bones.

Midfoot ulcers that result from increased plantar pressure over the rocker bottom deformity heal more slowly than ulcers on the forefoot.

Performing the Semmes-Weinstein test

In the Semmes-Weinstein test, the practitioner uses a special monofilament to assess protective sensation in the feet of a patient with diabetes. This test helps to identify the degree of sensory neuropathy.

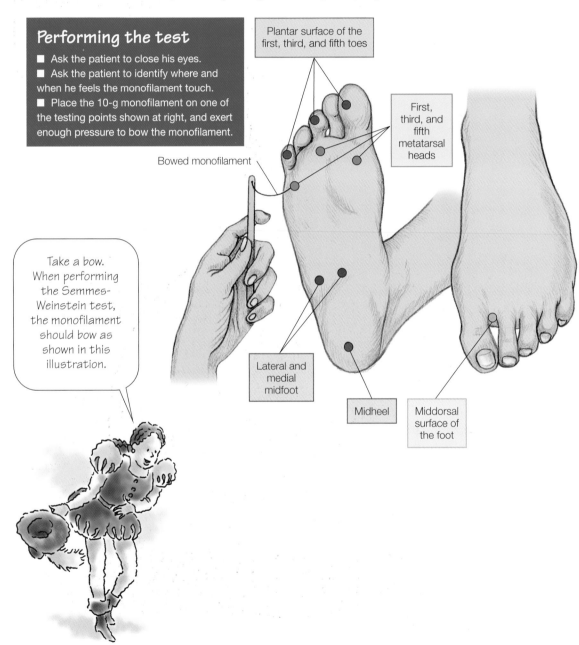

Performing the test

■ Ask the patient to close his eyes.
■ Ask the patient to identify where and when he feels the monofilament touch.
■ Place the 10-g monofilament on one of the testing points shown at right, and exert enough pressure to bow the monofilament.

Plantar surface of the first, third, and fifth toes

First, third, and fifth metatarsal heads

Bowed monofilament

Take a bow. When performing the Semmes-Weinstein test, the monofilament should bow as shown in this illustration.

Lateral and medial midfoot

Midheel

Middorsal surface of the foot

Characteristics

Diabetic foot ulcers commonly develop under a bony prominence, such as the one shown here under the metatarsal head of the great toe.

Impaired circulation and sensory neuropathy set the stage for ulcers to develop. These conditions allow excessive, repetitive pressure on the soles of the feet to go unchecked, commonly leading to an ulcer.

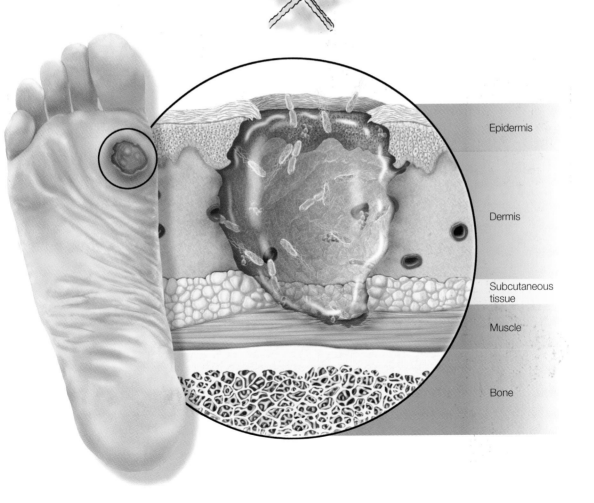

Epidermis

Dermis

Subcutaneous tissue

Muscle

Bone

Characteristics of skin surrounding a diabetic foot ulcer

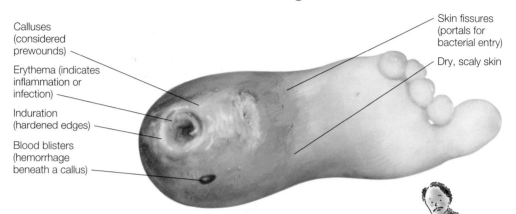

Calluses (considered prewounds)

Erythema (indicates inflammation or infection)

Induration (hardened edges)

Blood blisters (hemorrhage beneath a callus)

Skin fissures (portals for bacterial entry)

Dry, scaly skin

take note

Documenting a diabetic foot ulcer

2/28/11	1430	Dressing changed on diabetic foot ulcer on (L)heel.
		Ulcer measures 2 cm length, 3 cm width, 0.5 cm
		depth. No drainage or odor noted. Pedal pulses
		palpable. Site cleaned with NSS and allowed to dry
		thoroughly. Wound bed appears moist and pink with
		a thin ring of yellow slough at edges. Calloused border
		noted at wound edge from 6 o'clock to 8 o'clock.
		Hydrogel applied to site and dressed per physician
		order. Maintaining heels off bed, using blankets to
		elevate Pt. Ambulated with special orthotic shoe
		to off-load pressure. Tolerated procedure well;
		rates pain as 1 on a 0-to-10 scale before and after
		procedure. ——————————— Diane Bettick, R.N.

Ulcer location	Characteristics
Plantar surface	Even wound margins
Great toe	Deep wound bed
Metatarsal head	Dry or low to moderate exudate
Heel	Low to moderate exudate
Tip or top of toe	Pale granulation tissue with ischemia or bright red, friable granulation tissue with infection

A closer look at diabetic foot ulcers

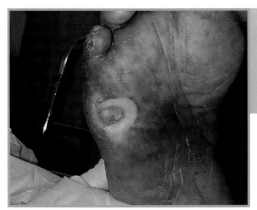

This photo shows a diabetic foot ulcer on the plantar surface of the fifth metatarsal head. The circular shape of the wound is consistent with a wound created by pressure over a bony prominence.

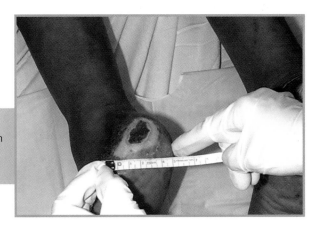

This photo shows a pressure ulcer that has developed over the heel from impaired protective sensation and poor mobility.

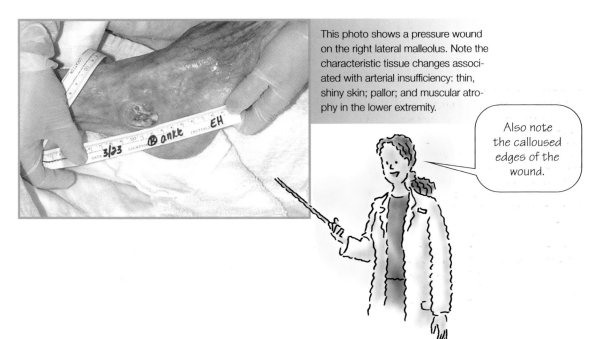

This photo shows a pressure wound on the right lateral malleolus. Note the characteristic tissue changes associated with arterial insufficiency: thin, shiny skin; pallor; and muscular atrophy in the lower extremity.

Also note the calloused edges of the wound.

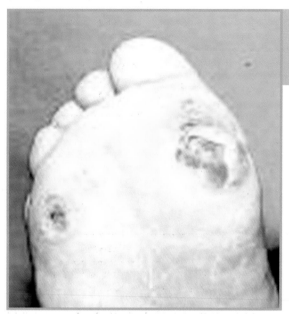

Ulcerations appear at the first and fifth metatarsal heads on this foot affected by Charcot's disease. Note the rocker bottom deformity.

Diabetic foot ulcers typically occur at sites of pressure, as in this heel ulcer.

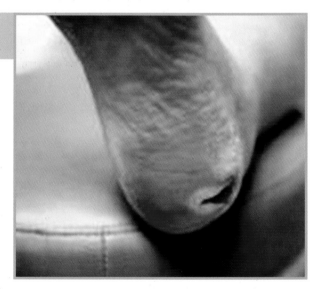

Classification

Depending on the classification system, diabetic foot ulcers are classified according to depth, presence of ischemia, and presence of infection.

> Classifying diabetic ulcers helps ensure that all members of the health care team provide treatment appropriate to the ulcer's severity.

University of Texas Diabetic Foot Classification System

The University of Texas Diabetic Foot Classification System provides a detailed categorization, which includes infection and ischemia.

Stage	Grade 0	Grade I	Grade II	Grade III
A	Preulcerative or post-ulcerative foot at risk for further ulceration	Superficial ulcer without tendon, capsule, or bone involvement	Ulcer penetrating to tendon or joint capsule	Ulcer penetrating to bone
B	Presence of infection	Presence of infection	Presence of infection	Presence of infection
C	Presence of ischemia	Presence of ischemia	Presence of ischemia	Presence of ischemia
D	Presence of infection and ischemia	Presence of infection and ischemia	Presence of infection and ischemia	Presence of infection and ischemia

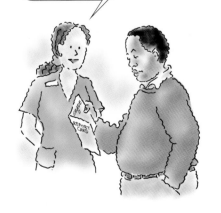

> This isn't like in school. In this instance, a low score is a good thing.

Wagner Ulcer Grade Classification

In the Wagner Ulcer Grade Classification, less-complex ulcers receive lower scores; more-complex ulcers, higher scores. Ulcers with higher scores may require surgical intervention or amputation.

Grade	Characteristics
0	▪ Preulcerous lesion ▪ Healed ulcer ▪ Presence of bony deformity
1	▪ Superficial ulcer without subcutaneous tissue involvement
2	▪ Penetration through the subcutaneous tissue; may expose bone, tendon, ligament, or joint capsule
3	▪ Osteitis, abscess, or osteomyelitis
4	▪ Gangrene of a digit
5	▪ Gangrene requiring foot amputation

Treatment

Successful ulcer healing depends on proper wound care and off-loading. The care plan may also include debridement, antimicrobials, biotherapies, and surgery.

Treatment algorithm for diabetic ulcers

- Establish etiology.
- Review past medical treatments.
- Review medication history.
- Perform noninvasive vascular assessment.
- Evaluate the patient's footwear.

Ischemic: Ankle-brachial index < 0.8
Vascular consult (if indicated)

Neuropathic: Ankle-brachial index > 0.9
Assess degree of neuropathy

Debridement

Ischemic, stable
- Nonaggressive dressing treatment

Nonischemic, neuropathic
- Debride hyperkeratotic rim
- Perform aggressive sharp debridement

Infection?

Yes   No   Yes

Localized soft tissue
- Broad-spectrum oral antibiotics
- Reevaluation in 1 week
- Non-weight-bearing activity (if possible)
- Control of diabetes

Wound care

Localized bone; systemic
- Admission to hospital
- Appropriate cultures
- I.V. antibiotics
- Possibly, surgical intervention

Wound care algorithm for diabetic ulcers

```
Evaluate patient.
        ↓
Evaluate footwear.
        ↓
Surgical referral for bony deformities
```

Wagner Grade 0	Wagner Grade 1	Wagner Grade 2	Wagner Grade 3	Wagner Grades 4 and 5
■ Padding and accommodative devices ■ Callus debridement	■ Follow Grade 0 protocol ■ Topical silver sulfadiazine (Silvadene) on highly contaminated wounds ■ Nonocclusive dressing ■ Weekly evaluation until healed ■ Plantar surface—gauze dressing ■ Dorsal surface—occlusive or nonocclusive dressing ■ Growth factor (becaplermin [Regranex]) when ankle-brachial index is > 0.45	■ Follow Grade 1 protocol ■ Rule out osteomyelitis (X-ray, bone scan, bone biopsy, or MRI) ■ Non-weight-bearing activity ■ Surgical consult ■ Plantar surface—gauze, amorphous hydrogel, alginate, or foam dressing ■ Dorsal surface—occlusive dressing ■ Topical antimicrobial cream, ointment, or amorphous hydrogel ■ Growth factor (becaplermin [Regranex]) when ankle-brachial index is > 0.45	■ Follow Grade 1 protocol ■ Rule out osteomyelitis (X-ray, bone scan, bone biopsy, or MRI) ■ Plantar surface—gauze, amorphous hydrogel, alginate, or foam dressing ■ Dorsal surface—nonocclusive dressing ■ Topical antimicrobial cream, ointment, or amorphous hydrogel	■ Surgical consult and intervention

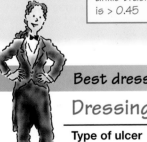

Best dressed

Dressings for diabetic foot ulcers

Type of ulcer	Recommended dressings
Dry	■ Hydrogel
Wet	■ Alginate ■ Foam ■ Collagen
Shallow	■ Transparent film ■ Hydrocolloid
Tunneling or deep	■ Alginate ropes (for wet ulcers) ■ Hydrogel impregnated gauze (for dry ulcers)
Infected	■ Iodosorb (a gel that cleans the wound by absorbing fluid, exudate, and bacteria) ■ Acticoat or Arglaes (products with an antimicrobial component)
Bleeding	■ Alginate

Off-loading

Patients with diabetic neuropathy no longer feel the pain that normally precedes tissue damage. Therefore, relieving pressure from plantar tissues—known as *off-loading*—is key to treating and preventing ulcers. Off-loading can be accomplished using nonsurgical and surgical interventions.

Nonsurgical interventions

■ Therapeutic footwear (possibly with rocker soles)

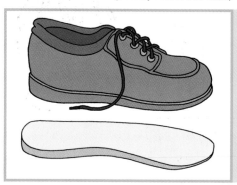

This shoe has a toe box with extra depth and width to accommodate bony deformities, such as claw toes and hallux valgus (displacement of the great toe toward other toes). The shoe can also be modified to allow room for a widened hindfoot. The soft, thick inlay provides comfort and protection.

■ Custom orthotics
■ Walking casts (such as a total contact cast)
■ Walkers
■ Splints

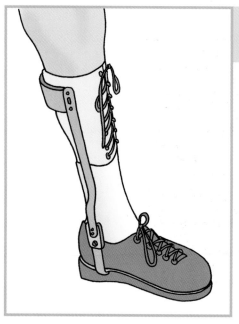

This ankle-foot orthosis is used to relieve pressure from the heel.

Surgical interventions

■ Exostectomy
■ Digital arthroplasty
■ Bone and joint resections
■ Partial calcanectomy

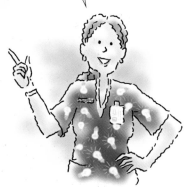

Keep in mind that using an off-loading device can increase the patient's risk of falling. Be sure to teach the patient about fall prevention.

Prevention

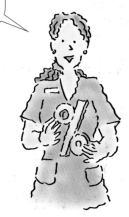

Comprehensive foot care programs can reduce ulcer-related amputation rates by up to 50%.

Diabetic ulcer prevention starts with teaching patients how to control diabetes and how to care for their feet.

Teaching topic	Teaching tips
Diabetes control	• Emphasize the importance of controlling diabetes. Discuss the consequences of failing to control diabetes (such as peripheral neuropathy and vascular damage). • Explain that careful glycemic control (by monitoring Hb A_{1c} levels at regular intervals) can reduce the frequency and severity of neuropathy in people with type 1 or type 2 diabetes.
Foot hygiene	• Check feet daily for injury or pressure areas (using a long-handled mirror may make viewing easier). • Wash feet with a mild soap, and dry thoroughly between the toes. • Before getting in, check bath water to make sure it isn't too hot. (Test the water with an elbow, use a thermometer, or ask a family member to help.) • Apply a moisturizing cream to feet to prevent dry, cracked skin and to balance skin pH. Don't apply moisturizer between the toes. • Cut toenails off squarely. Consult a podiatrist if toenails are deformed and thickened. • Don't go barefooted; the risk of injury is too great.
Choosing socks	• Use silver ion–lined socks for fungus control, if needed. • Wear white or light-colored socks to make bleeding from trauma easy to detect. • Wear natural fiber socks (which breathe better than synthetics). • Choose socks that wick perspiration away from the feet (such as cotton-blended socks) to prevent maceration. • Use diabetic padded socks for shear and friction control.
Choosing shoes	• Wear shoes that fit well, not shoes that are too tight or loose. • Wear shoes that breathe to reduce maceration and fungal infections. • Wear new shoes for short periods (less than 1 hour) each day initially; gradually increase the time as your feet adjust. • If you have any foot deformities or have a history of ulceration, wear professionally fitted shoes. • If possible, wash your shoes to destroy microorganisms. • Check your shoes before putting them on to make sure they don't contain anything that could cause an injury.

VISION QUEST

Show and tell

Describe the pathophysiology of sensory neuropathy illustrated here.

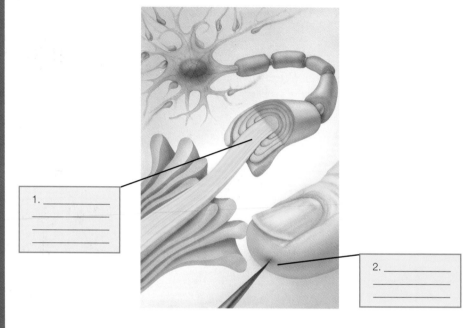

1. _____
   _____
   _____

2. _____
   _____
   _____

Able to label?

Identify the bony abnormalities associated with diabetic motor neuropathy on this illustration.

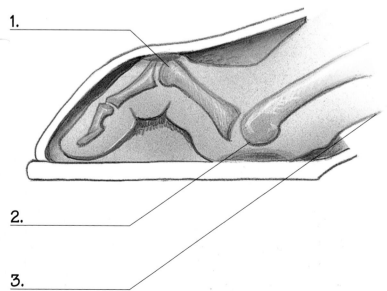

1. _____

2. _____

3. _____

Answers: Show and tell 1. Ischemia or demyelination causes nerve death or deterioration, 2. Decreased pain sensation results; Able to label? 1. Clawed toes, 2. Downward displacement of the metatarsal heads, 3. Increased arch height.

9
Malignant wounds

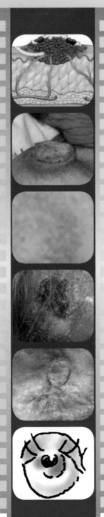

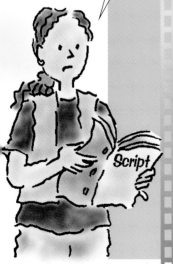

Talk about a sad story! Malignant wounds set the stage for a number of challenges for both the patient and the caregiver.

Script

Causes

Malignant wounds develop when a primary or metastatic tumor infiltrates the epidermis. Occurring in 6% to 10% of cancer patients, these wounds grow rapidly and commonly invade surrounding tissues and organs, sometimes creating sinus tracts and fistulas. Having a cauliflower-like appearance, malignant wounds are poorly perfused with friable, fragile blood vessels and contain large amounts of necrotic tissue.

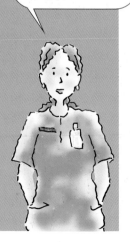

Malignant wounds most commonly occur in patients with breast cancer. However, they can also occur in patients with cancer of the head, neck, chest, and abdomen as well as in those with leukemia, lymphoma, and melanoma.

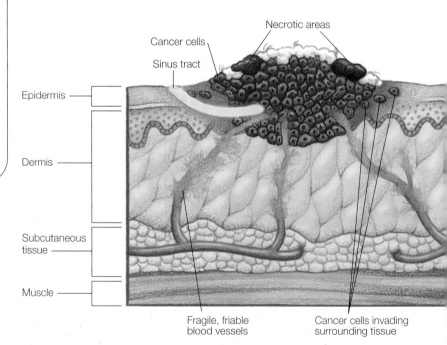

Necrotic areas

Cancer cells

Sinus tract

Epidermis

Dermis

Subcutaneous tissue

Muscle

Fragile, friable blood vessels

Cancer cells invading surrounding tissue

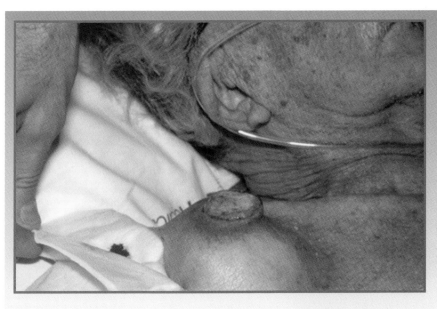

◄ This squamous cell carcinoma, after being neglected, ulcerated to form the malignant wound shown here.

This basal cell carcinoma was also neglected. It eventually ulcerated and invaded deeper tissue. ▶

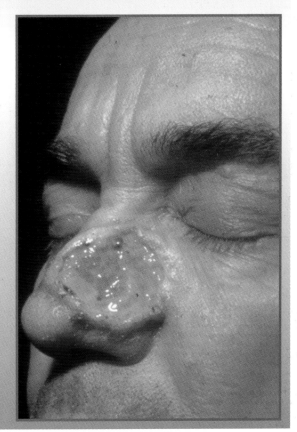

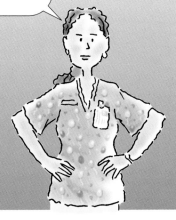

Malignant wounds can develop from a skin cancer that has been neglected.

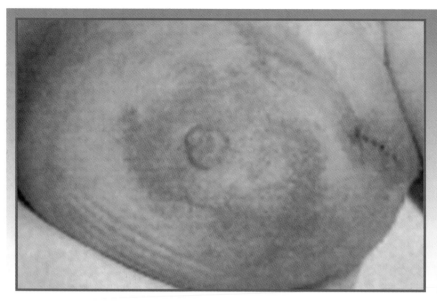

◄ This photo shows an inflamed carcinoma of the breast.

The malignant wound shown here resulted when a lymphoma metastasized to the patient's scalp. ►

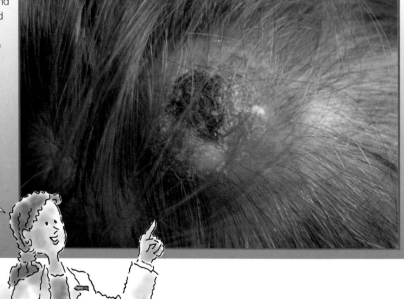

When a primary tumor outgrows its blood supply, it can invade the skin, resulting in a malignant wound.

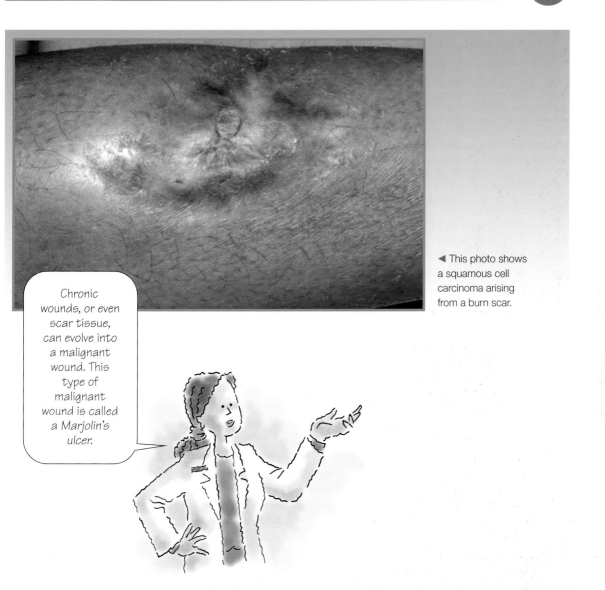

◀ This photo shows a squamous cell carcinoma arising from a burn scar.

Chronic wounds, or even scar tissue, can evolve into a malignant wound. This type of malignant wound is called a Marjolin's ulcer.

Complications

Problem	Causes	Management strategies
Odor	Nonviable, necrotic tissue and excessive drainage create an ideal environment for bacterial growth. In turn, this produces a foul odor. Odor-causing aerobic bacteria include Klebsiella, Proteus, Pseudomonas, and Staphylococcus. Anaerobic bacterial causes include Clostridium and *Bacteroides fragilis*.	• Change dressings and gently irrigate the wound with normal saline solution at frequent intervals. • Apply topical antibiotics to reduce the amount of bacteria. • Use other topical antimicrobials, such as metronidazole gel (MetroGel), crushed metronidazole tablets, or silver sulfadiazine (Silvadene), as indicated. • Use charcoal dressings, such as CarboFlex and Actisorb Plus. • Apply mentholatum (Vicks VapoRub) near the patient's or caregiver's nostrils to minimize the perception of odor. • Place a tray of kitty litter, baking soda, or charcoal under the patient's bed to absorb odors. • Apply a pouching system to the wound to help control odors.
Bleeding	Malignant cells secrete tissue permeability factor, which increases vascular permeability and promotes a loss of protein and fibrinogen. This causes the blood vessels surrounding a malignant wound to become friable and fragile, and the blood to have an impaired ability to clot.	• Use nonadherent dressings (such as silicone dressings) to minimize tissue trauma and reduce the risk of bleeding. • Avoid frequent or unnecessary dressing changes. • Apply sucralfate (Carafate) suspension or paste to the surface of friable blood vessels to provide barrier protection. • Assist with surgical intervention (cauterization) or the application of topical epinephrine (Adrenalin) 1:1000 to control profuse bleeding. • Apply silver nitrate sticks or topical thrombin (Thrombin-JMI) to control sudden, profuse bleeding. • Administer oral antifibrinolytics (such as tranexamic acid [Cyklokapron]), as prescribed, to control severe bleeding.
Exudate (drainage)	The leakage of fibrinogen and plasma colloids by vessels in the wound causes exudate to form. Bacteria in the wound release enzymes that liquefy tissue, producing additional exudate.	• Use highly absorbent dressings (such as calcium alginate, foam, and hydrofiber) in wounds with moderate to large amounts of exudate. • Administer topical or systemic antimicrobials, as prescribed, to reduce bacterial load and exudate. • Use a wound drainage system, such as a pouch, on wounds with large amounts of exudate. (Avoid using a negative pressure system.) • Protect the surrounding skin from maceration and irritation.
Pruritus (itching)	As malignant cells invade surrounding tissue, the skin stretches and the peripheral nerves become irritated, commonly resulting in pruritus. Fungal infections may also cause pruritus.	• Chill hydrogel sheet dressings in the refrigerator and then apply to the wound. • Apply menthol creams to the affected area. • Advise the patient to use cool or lukewarm water to bathe or shower, rather than hot water. • Tell the patient to use a cool mist humidifier during colder months. • Advise the patient that antihistamines typically have no effect on the pruritus associated with malignant wounds.
Pain	Pressure on nerve endings from the tumor as well as exposure of the dermis to air may cause chronic pain. Dressing changes and other procedures may also worsen pain.	• Use a reliable and valid pain assessment tool—such as the visual analog, numeric pain intensity, or FACES pain-rating scales—to accurately assess the patient's level of pain. • Administer prescribed pain medication or topical anesthetics as ordered and before changing dressings or performing procedures.

Treatment

The goal behind any wound management system is to protect the wound and the surrounding areas and to provide an ideal environment for healing. However, because malignant wounds tend to occur near the end of a patient's life, treatment typically focuses on controlling symptoms and offering psychological support rather than on healing.

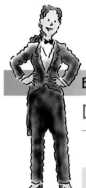

Best dressed

Dressings used for malignant wounds

Wound characteristics	Dressings	Medications
Exudate	▪ Foam ▪ Calcium alginates ▪ Hydrofibers ▪ Mesalt	▪ Antibiotic creams
Odor	▪ Foam ▪ Calcium alginates ▪ Hydrofibers ▪ Composite ▪ Charcoal ▪ Occlusive	▪ Topical metronidazole ▪ Antibiotic creams
Pain	▪ Hydrogels (if wound has minimal drainage) ▪ Foam ▪ Calcium alginates ▪ Hydrofibers ▪ Nonadhesive	▪ Topical anesthetics ▪ Oral or parenteral pain medications
Bleeding	▪ Foam ▪ Hydrofibers ▪ Hemostatic (such as Gelfoam, Spongostan, and Oxycel)	▪ Topical epinephrine (use with caution) ▪ Silver nitrate (to cauterize bleeding)

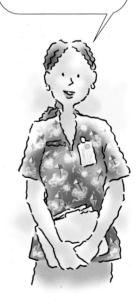

Because it's easier to control drainage, odor, and bleeding in a small wound, chemotherapy and radiation treatments are sometimes used to reduce the size of a malignant wound.

VISION QUEST

Matchmaker

Match the five complications of malignant wounds shown on the left with the management strategies shown on the right.

1. Odor _____
2. Bleeding _____
3. Exudate _____
4. Pruritus _____
5. Pain _____

A. Administer analgesics as ordered.
B. Use nonadherent dressings.
C. Apply topical antimicrobials to the wound.
D. Use a wound drainage system such as a pouch.
E. Apply cooled hydrogel sheets to the wound.

Rebus riddle

Sound out each group of symbols and letters to reveal the disease most likely to give rise to a malignant wound.

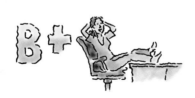 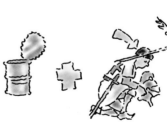

Answers: Matchmaker 1. C, 2. B, 3. D, 4. E, 5. A; Rebus riddle Breast cancer.

10
Atypical wounds

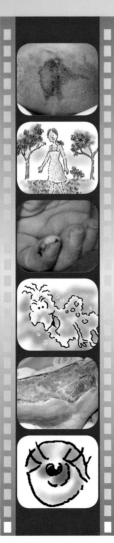

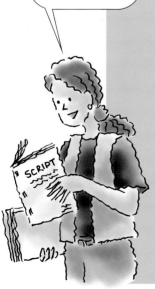

Now here's a script I can get excited about! It's got a very unusual storyline.

Causes

External or traumatic causes	Inflammatory processes	Infection
■ Bites ■ Burns ■ Radiation ■ Stings	■ Pyoderma gangrenosum ■ Vasculitis	■ Atypical mycobacteria ■ Deep fungal infections

Metabolic and genetic disorders	Neoplasms	Vasculopathies
■ Calciphylaxis ■ Epidermolysis bullosa ■ Sickle cell anemia	■ Basal cell carcinoma ■ Kaposi's sarcoma ■ Lymphoma ■ Squamous cell carcinoma	■ Antiphospholipid antibody syndrome ■ Cryoglobulinemia ■ Cryofibrinogenemia

Types

Bites

Bites, such as those from insects and animals, are one type of atypical wound.

Erythematous lesion with central eschar caused by a spider bite

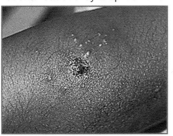

Wounds from several dog bites

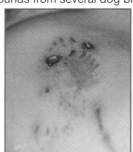

Intertrigo

Intertrigo is the inflammation of a skinfold or two areas of skin that rub together.

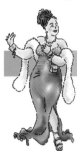

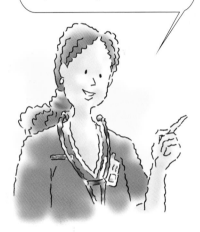

> Intertrigo can occur in any skinfold but is most prevalent under the breasts, in the pannus (abdominal skinfolds), and in the axillary, submaxillary, groin, and perineal areas.

Special attention

Intertrigo in bariatric patients

Bariatric patients are at higher risk for developing intertriginous dermatitis (dermatitis that occurs between skinfolds) because multiple large skinfolds create conditions that are perfect for infection and inflammation. These conditions include:

- pressure of large skinfolds on underlying skin, creating pressure-induced injury
- moisture (perspiration is trapped under skinfolds, resulting in maceration)
- friction
- shear with movement, resulting in fissures
- physical challenges in maintaining hygiene
- warm, dark, moist conditions that favor the growth of yeast and fungi.

Intravenous extravasation ulcers

Extravasation is the unintentional administration of a vesicant solution into surrounding tissue. Vesicants (chemotherapy agents, certain electrolyte solutions, radiographic contrast media, and vasopressors) are solutions capable of causing tissue injury or destruction if they escape into surrounding tissue.

Chronic ulceration from chemotherapy infiltration

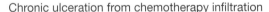

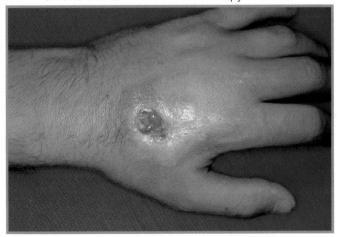

Necrotizing fasciitis

Necrotizing fasciitis is a severe type of infection in which bacteria enter the body through a minor wound and release harmful toxins that interfere with the tissue's blood supply.

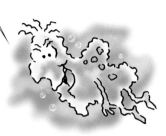

Once my friends and I spread, necrotizing fasciitis can quickly lead to death.

Stages

Tenderness, warm skin, and a painful bump or spot on the skin

Quick formation of a bronze or purple-colored blister

Tissue necrosis, with gangrening of the area

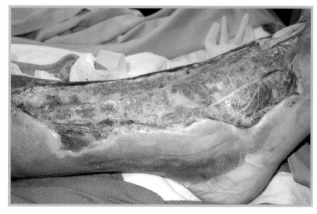

Pyoderma gangrenosum ulcers

Pyoderma gangrenosum ulcers most commonly occur on the legs after injury or trauma. Multiple ulcers in one area sometimes merge into one large ulcer.

Painful, open ulcer with reddish-purple irregular borders

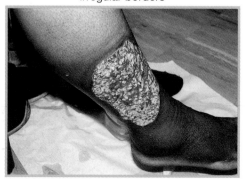

Scleroderma

In scleroderma, cutaneous lesions usually occur on the hands, face, neck, and upper chest.

Acrocyanosis and ulcer formation in scleroderma

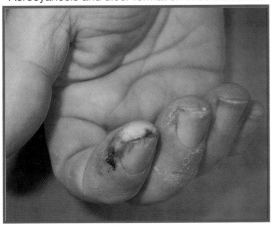

Systemic lupus erythematosus ulcers

Systemic lupus erythematosus (SLE) ulcers most commonly occur on the scalp and face and sometimes look like psoriasis.

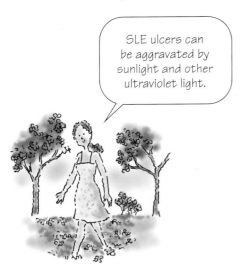

SLE ulcers can be aggravated by sunlight and other ultraviolet light.

Red, scaly SLE ulcer

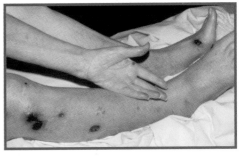

Thromboangiitis obliterans

Also known as *Buerger's disease*, thromboangiitis obliterans is inflammatory thrombosis that can occur in some superficial veins and small and medium-sized arteries. It causes arterial ischemia in distal extremities and superficial thrombophlebitis.

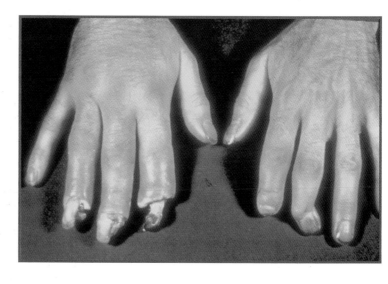

Warfarin-induced necrosis

Warfarin (Coumadin)–induced necrosis commonly occurs on the breasts, buttocks, thighs, and abdomen.

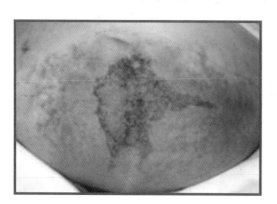

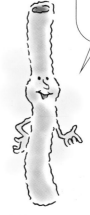

The abundance of small dermal blood vessels in fatty tissue may explain why warfarin-induced necrosis is more common in some areas.

Treatments

Black widow spider bite
- Immediate medical attention
- Cool compresses
- Elevation, if possible
- Antivenom
- Calcium gluconate
- Antihistamines
- Analgesics
- Local wound care

Brown recluse spider bite
- Cool compresses
- Elevation, if possible
- Analgesics
- Systemic corticosteroids
- Aggressive local wound care
- Debridement
- Grafting

Dog bite
- Antibiotics
- Rabies therapy
- Tetanus vaccination
- Aggressive local wound care
- Debridement and grafting, if the wound is extensive

Intertrigo
- Eliminating friction, heat, and maceration by keeping skin folds cool and dry
- Antimycotic agents (miconazole, clotrimazole)
- Protective barrier creams such as Triple paste and Desitin

I.V. extravasation ulcers
- Immediate cessation of the infusion
- Flushing of the area with normal saline solution within 24 hours
- Local infiltration of the affected area with dilute antidote (varies depending on the drug extravasated)
- Debridement and topical care, depending on wound characteristics
- Grafting
- Possible amputation, if gangrene results

Necrotizing fasciitis
- Frequent surgical debridement
- Broad-spectrum antibiotics
- Grafting or flap
- Aggressive local wound care
- Negative-pressure wound therapy
- Local wound care

Pyoderma gangrenosum ulcers
- Systemic management of underlying disease
- Corticosteroids (topical, systemic, intralesional)
- Immunosuppressive agents such as cyclosporine (systemic, topical)
- Antimicrobial agents, such as tetracycline and vancomycin
- Anti–tumor necrosis factor (alpha) medications, such as infliximab (Remicade) and etanercept (Enbrel)
- Blood products
- Immunomodulators, such as I.V. immunoglobulin (IVIG)
- Hyperbaric oxygen
- Aggressive local wound care (such as with foams, gels, and silver dressings)

Scleroderma
- Systemic management of underlying disease
- Nitrates, such as nitroglycerin, for vasodilation
- Debridement
- Hyperbaric oxygen
- Local wound care (commonly treated like vascular wounds)

SLE ulcers
- Systemic management of underlying disease
- Corticosteroids (systemic, topical)
- Immunosuppressants (such as azathioprine [Imuran] or cyclophosphamide [Cytoxan])
- Hyperbaric oxygen
- Local wound care

Thromboangiitis obliterans
- Smoking abstinence (cornerstone of treatment)
- Calcium channel blockers such as nifedipine (Procardia)
- Arterial bypass
- Major or minor amputations
- Avoidance of cold temperatures
- Aspirin
- Vasodilators
- Surgical sympathectomy for pain management

Warfarin (Coumadin)-induced necrosis
- Discontinuation of warfarin
- I.V. heparin
- Debridement
- Grafting
- Muscle flaps

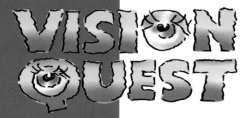

VISION QUEST

Matchmaker

Match the atypical wounds shown at right with their names.

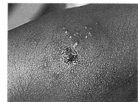 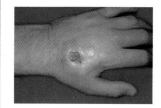 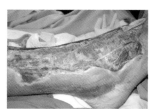

1. _____ 2. _____ 3. _____

A. Necrotizing fasciitis
B. Spider bite
C. Intravenous extravasation ulcer

My word!

Use the clues to help you unscramble three terms related to atypical wounds. Then use the circled letters to answer the question posed.

Question: Intertrigo is the term used to describe inflammation of a what?

1. A brand name for warfarin

aimnocud _Ο__ _Ο__

2. Type of anemia that is one cause of atypical wounds

kslice lecl Ο__Ο__ ___Ο

3. Type of infection in which bacteria release toxins that interfere with the tissue's blood supply

zircontinge isifcatis Ο_____Ο__Ο_

Answer: _____

Answers: Matchmaker 1. C, 2. B, 3. A; My word! 1. Coumadin, 2. Sickle cell, 3. Necrotizing fasciitis; Question: Skinfold.

11

Wound care products

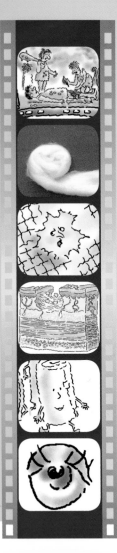

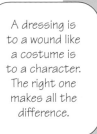

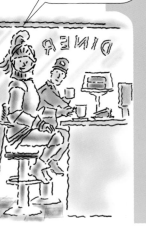

A dressing is to a wound like a costume is to a character. The right one makes all the difference.

Development of wound care products

Over time, wound care has evolved from a fairly rudimentary practice that focused primarily on the injury to a process that takes the patient's overall health into account.

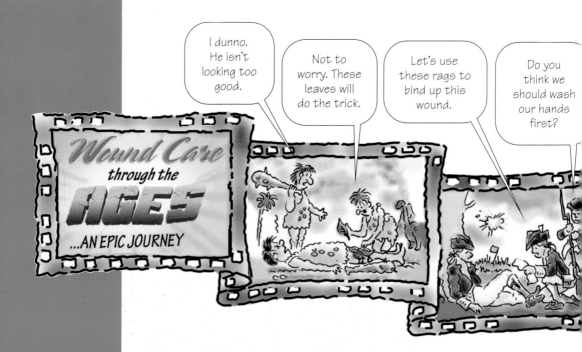

Dressings

Selecting the right dressing for a wound means taking into account:
- the size of the wound
- the amount of moisture in the wound
- whether the wound is infected
- the condition of the surrounding skin.

> Controlling the amount of moisture in a wound is crucial to the healing process. That's why dressings are commonly classified according to whether they add moisture to a wound bed or whether they absorb it.

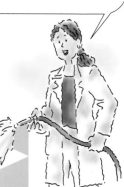

Dressing moisture scale

Use this chart to quickly determine the category of dressing that's appropriate for your patient.

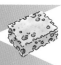

Absorb moisture		Neutral (maintain existing moisture level)		Add moisture	
☐ Alginates	☐ Foams	■ Composites	■ Transparent films	■ Sheet hydrogels	☐ Amorphous hydrogels
☐ Specialty absorptives	☐ Hydrocolloids		■ Biologicals		
☐ Gauze	☐ Wound fillers		■ Collagen dressings		
			■ Contact layers		

> Keep in mind that new wound care products are being developed all the time, while old products are being improved. Make sure you stay up-to-date on all the "new releases."

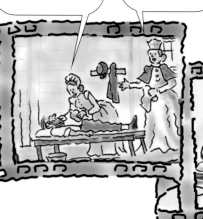

> This iodine-treated gauze is the greatest thing since sliced bread.

> Um, sliced bread hasn't been invented yet.

> Hmm...This patient is malnourished and has diabetes. That will definitely influence how I treat this wound.

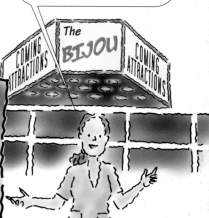

The BIJOU

Alginate dressings

Made from seaweed, alginate dressings are available as sterile pads, ribbons, or ropes. These nonocclusive dressings are nonadherent and promote autolytic debridement to soften and remove necrotic tissue.

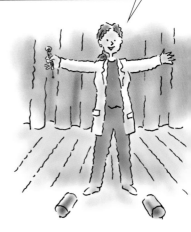

And now, I'm proud to introduce the cast of characters in our wound care epic. In alphabetical order—beginning with alginate dressings and ending with wound fillers—let's hear it for the dressings of today!

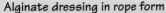
Alginate dressing in rope form

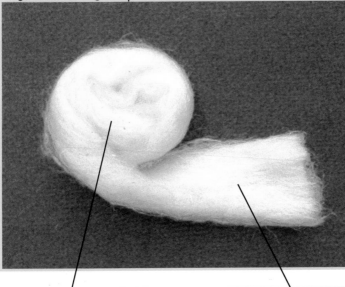

Very soft, nonwoven fibers turn into a biodegradable gel as they absorb exudate.

Fibers encourage hemostasis in minimally bleeding wounds.

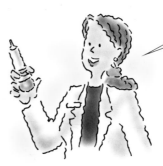

To facilitate dressing removal—and to make dressing changes less painful—saturate the dressing with normal saline solution before removal. Use additional saline to clean the wound of any remaining dressing fibers.

Antimicrobial dressings

Antimicrobial dressings contain ingredients such as silver, iodine, and polyhexethylene to protect against bacteria. Available in various forms—including transparent dressings, gauze, island dressings, foams, and absorptive fillers—some antimicrobial dressings also provide a moist environment for wound healing.

> Besides making beautiful jewelry, silver has powerful antimicrobial and bactericidal properties. In fact, it's been used for centuries to prevent and treat infection.

> Silver in the dressing attacks bacteria and helps bind toxins.

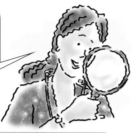

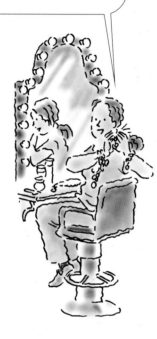

Silver-impregnated antimicrobial dressing

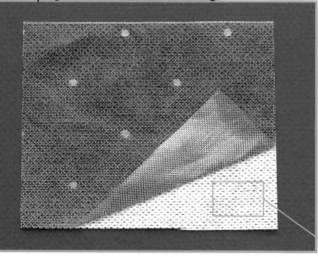

Silver-impregnated activated charcoal cloth

Silver ions

Bacteria

Bacteria leaking fluid as it dies

How antimicrobial dressings work

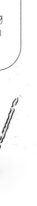

Signs of wound infection include redness, swelling, and increased pain. If that isn't bad enough, infection can stop the healing process and worsen wound breakdown.

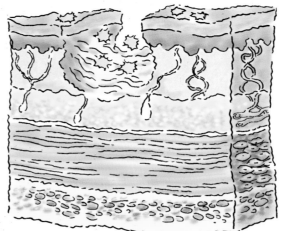

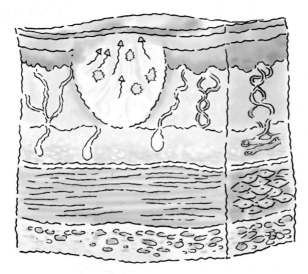

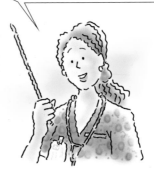

Once applied, an antimicrobial dressing immediately begins to release silver in a controlled fashion. The silver destroys bacteria in the dressing and the wound. Many antimicrobial dressings also absorb drainage and help keep the wound moist for optimum healing.

Collagen dressings

Made with bovine or avian collagen, collagen dressings are available in sheets, pads, particles, and gels.

Collagen dressings encourage wound healing by stimulating the deposit of collagen fibers necessary for the growth of tissue and blood vessels.

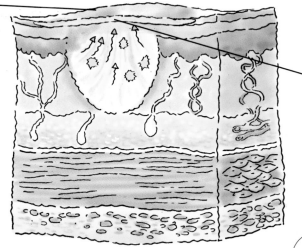

These highly absorbent dressings also maintain a moist wound environment.

Collagen in particle form

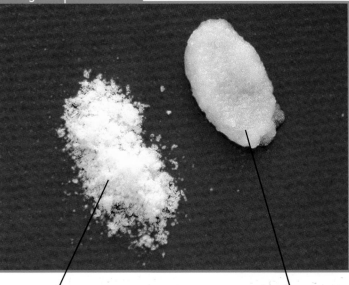

Make sure wound infection has been treated and necrotic tissue debrided before using a collagen dressing.

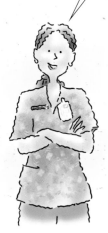

Some bovine collagen is processed into fine particles, as shown here. These particles can then be shaken into a wound bed.

Mixing with moist exudate in the wound, the particles gel as they absorb many times their weight in excess fluid.

Composite dressings

Composite dressings combine two or more types of dressings into one. Typical layers include:

1 Waterproof, vapor-permeable film

2 Absorbent foam layer

3 Silicone inner layer

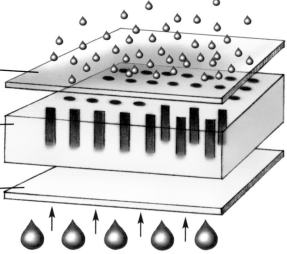

By combining two or more materials into one dressing, composite dressings reduce confusion and make dressing changes a snap.

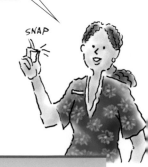

SNAP

A closer look at a composite dressing

This composite dressing stimulates autolytic debridement while controlling moisture.

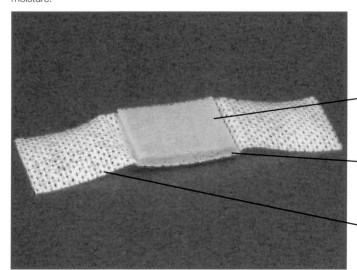

A thin, transparent, semipermeable film allows the exchange of gas and water vapor while blocking bacteria.

A highly absorbent foam-type matrix slowly releases ingredients that clean and moisturize the wound.

The adhesive backing consists of a breathable cloth.

Contact layer dressings

Made of woven or perforated material, contact layer dressings are single-layer dressings designed to lie directly on the wound's surface. A secondary dressing is then placed on top of the contact layer.

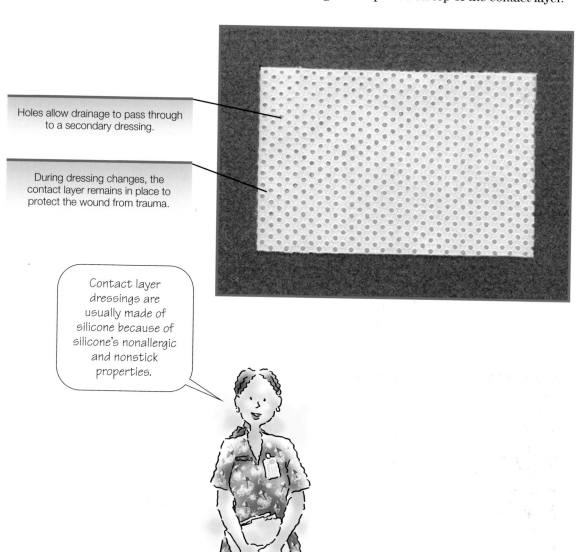

Holes allow drainage to pass through to a secondary dressing.

During dressing changes, the contact layer remains in place to protect the wound from trauma.

Contact layer dressings are usually made of silicone because of silicone's nonallergic and nonstick properties.

Foam dressings

Foam dressings are absorbent, spongelike polymer dressings. In addition to providing thermal insulation, they help create a moist wound environment.

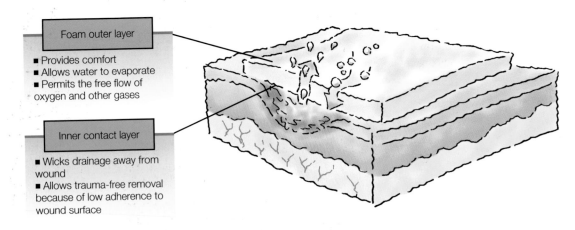

Foam outer layer

- Provides comfort
- Allows water to evaporate
- Permits the free flow of oxygen and other gases

Inner contact layer

- Wicks drainage away from wound
- Allows trauma-free removal because of low adherence to wound surface

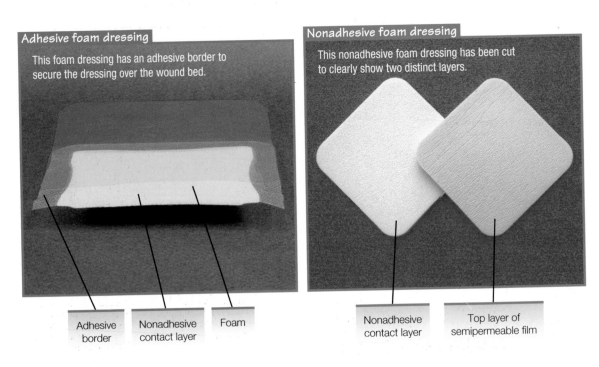

Adhesive foam dressing

This foam dressing has an adhesive border to secure the dressing over the wound bed.

Adhesive border

Nonadhesive contact layer

Foam

Nonadhesive foam dressing

This nonadhesive foam dressing has been cut to clearly show two distinct layers.

Nonadhesive contact layer

Top layer of semipermeable film

Hydrocolloid dressings

Made of a carbohydrate-based material, hydrocolloid dressings are adhesive, moldable wafers that are impermeable to oxygen, water, and water vapor. Besides being somewhat absorbent, these dressings help maintain a moist wound environment and promote autolytic debridement. These dressings are available in various thicknesses.

> Hydrocolloids turn to gel as they absorb moisture, making the dressing become spongy and lighter in color over the wound. Reassure the patient that this is normal and, by itself, doesn't necessitate a dressing change.

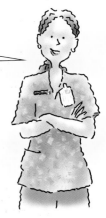

Hydrocolloid dressing

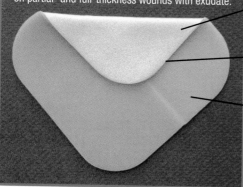

This dressing, which is 2 mm thick, would be used on partial- and full-thickness wounds with exudate.

The exterior surface protects the wound from outside contaminants.

The hydrocolloid layer turns to gel as hydrocolloids absorb moisture.

The adhesive layer adheres to the surrounding skin, but not the wound; adherence decreases as gel forms.

Thin hydrocolloid dressing

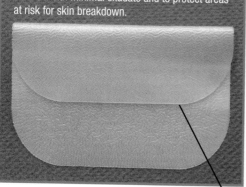

Thin hydrocolloid dressings are used on superficial wounds with minimal exudate and to protect areas at risk for skin breakdown.

The hydrocolloid interior of this dressing is less than 1 mm thick.

Hydrocolloid paste and gel

Hydrocolloids are also available in paste, powder, and gel forms. Pastes and gels require a secondary dressing, such as a hydrocolloid wafer.

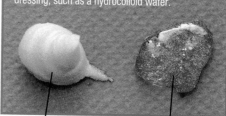

Hydrocolloid paste
- Used to manage dermal wounds with light drainage

Hydrocolloid gel
- Used on partial- and full-thickness wounds
- Fills dry wound cavities
- Promotes autolytic debridement

Hydrogel dressings

Made with a water or glycerin base, hydrogel dressings hydrate wounds and soften necrotic tissue. Because they contain a large percentage of water, these dressings provide limited absorption. Hydrogel dressings are available as a flexible sheet or a gel.

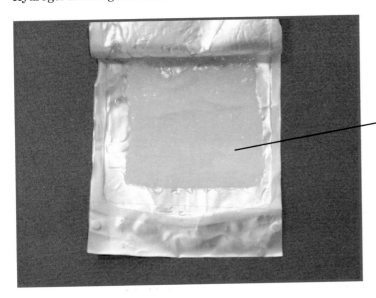

Hydrogel-impregnated gauze

- Hydrates wounds
- Softens necrotic tissue
- Cools and soothes burning wounds (such as skin tears and dermal wounds)

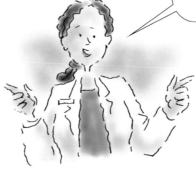

There's a good and bad side to every story. Although hydrogel dressings are great for hydrating wounds, they can also macerate the surrounding skin. Protect the healthy skin around the wound by applying a liquid film-forming dressing or protective ointment.

Amorphous hydrogels

Amorphous hydrogels are gels packaged in tubes. Depending on the components in the gel, amorphous hydrogels have a number of uses.

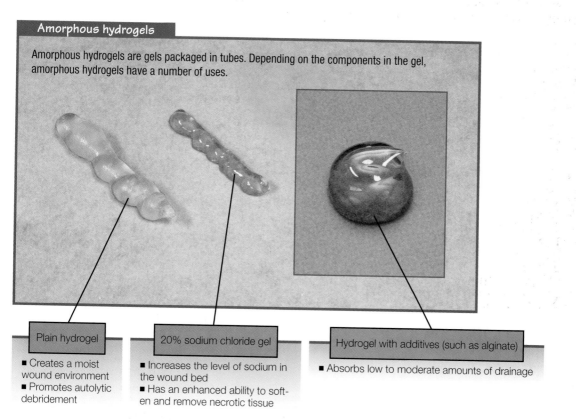

Plain hydrogel
- Creates a moist wound environment
- Promotes autolytic debridement

20% sodium chloride gel
- Increases the level of sodium in the wound bed
- Has an enhanced ability to soften and remove necrotic tissue

Hydrogel with additives (such as alginate)
- Absorbs low to moderate amounts of drainage

Specialty absorptive dressings

Specialty absorptive dressings, some with adhesive borders, contain multiple layers of a highly absorbent material, such as cotton or rayon. They're available as gels, pads, gauze, and pillows.

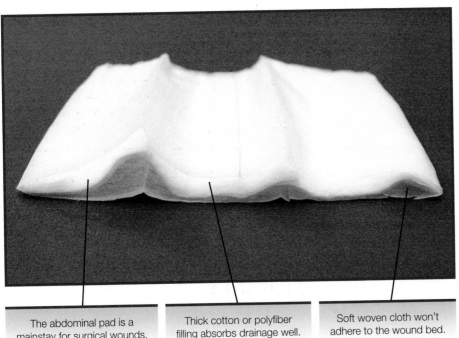

The abdominal pad is a mainstay for surgical wounds.

Thick cotton or polyfiber filling absorbs drainage well.

Soft woven cloth won't adhere to the wound bed.

Transparent film dressings

Made of polyurethane, transparent film dressings adhere to the skin and help maintain a moist wound environment. While these dressings are nonabsorbent, they promote autolytic debridement and stimulate the formation of granulation tissue.

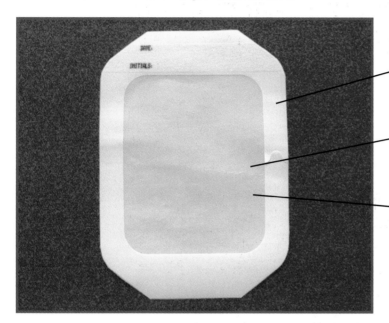

Backing is removed before application, leaving a clear, membranelike dressing.

Film allows the exchange of water vapor and oxygen while being impermeable to fluids and bacteria.

Transparent film allows visual inspection of the wound while the dressing is in place.

Wound fillers

Used to fill deep wounds, some wound fillers add moisture to the wound bed whereas others absorb drainage. Made of various materials, wound fillers are available as pastes, granules, strands, powders, beads, and gels.

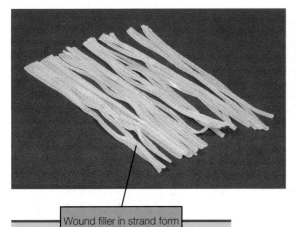

Wound filler in strand form

- Highly absorbent properties make it appropriate for wounds with heavy exudate.
- Strand form allows material to completely fill dead space.
- This particular filler contains silver, which has antimicrobial properties.

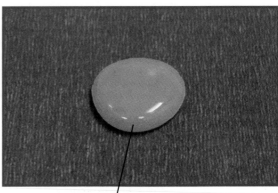

Wound filler in gel form

- Gel fills the wound evenly, helping prevent wound dehydration.
- Some gels effectively control wound odor.
- This dextrose-based gel mixes with wound drainage to coat and protect the wound and to provide a moist healing environment.

Wound care dressing review

Use this chart to quickly compare the various dressings, their indications for use, their advantages, and their disadvantages.

Dressing type	Indications for use	Advantages	Disadvantages
Alginates (Used as a primary dressing)	• Wounds with moderate to heavy drainage • Wounds with tunneling	• Hold up to 20 times their weight in fluid • May be cut to fit wound dimensions • May be layered for more absorption • Supplied in ropes for deep wound packing • Promote autolytic debridement	• May require irrigation for removal • Require secondary dressings • Can't be used on dry eschar or wounds with light drainage • May dehydrate dryer wounds
Antimicrobials (Used as a primary or secondary dressing)	• Infected wounds • Wounds with minimal to heavy drainage • Nonhealing wounds	• Help prevent or reduce infection • Effective against a broad spectrum of microorganisms	• May produce a hypersensitivity reaction in patients sensitive to silver or iodine • May sting when applied • May contribute to the development of resistant organisms (not yet known)
Biologicals (Used as a primary dressing)	• Ulcers (specific product used will vary according to ulcer thickness) • Skin graft donor sites • Burns	• Promote healing • Prevent infection and fluid loss • Ease discomfort	• May cause allergic reactions • May require secondary dressings
Collagens (Used as a primary dressing)	• Chronic, granulated wounds • Wounds with tunneling • Wounds with minimal to heavy drainage (depending upon specific product used)	• Available in various forms (gel, granules, and sheets; some also contain alginate) • Perform well on chronic, clean wounds • Conform well to wound bed • Are nonadherent	• May cause an allergic reaction in patients sensitive to collagen, bovine, or avian products • Require secondary dressings • Aren't appropriate for third-degree burns or wounds with dry beds

(continued)

Wound care dressing review *(continued)*

Dressing type	Indications for use	Advantages	Disadvantages
Composites (Used as a primary or secondary dressing)	▪ Wounds with minimal to heavy drainage ▪ Partial- to full-thickness wounds ▪ Wounds with granulation tissue, necrotic tissue, or both	▪ Available in various combinations, sizes, and shapes ▪ Conform well to wound bed ▪ Promote autolytic debridement	▪ May not provide a moist wound environment (depending on the product selected) and may dry the wound bed ▪ Can't be cut to fit without losing some dressing integrity ▪ Can't be used on third-degree burns ▪ Due to adhesive border, use may be limited if skin surrounding wound is fragile or nonintact
Contact layers (Used as a primary dressing)	▪ Partial- to full-thickness wounds ▪ Wounds with minimal to heavy drainage ▪ Skin graft donor sites	▪ Promote drainage to a secondary dressing while preventing the secondary dressing from adhering to the wound ▪ Minimize pain during dressing changes ▪ May be used with topical medications, fillers, or gauze dressings ▪ Can be cut to fit or overlap the wound's edges	▪ Require a secondary dressing ▪ Can't be used on stage I pressure ulcers, third-degree burns, infected wounds, and wounds with tunneling
Foams (Used as a primary or secondary dressing)	▪ Partial- to full-thickness wounds ▪ Wounds with minimal to heavy drainage (including around tubes)	▪ Nonadherent ▪ May be used alone (with an adhesive border) ▪ Can be used on infected wounds if changed daily ▪ May be used in combination with other products ▪ Wick moisture from the wound and allow evaporation (hydropolymer foam dressings)	▪ Without an adhesive border, may require a secondary dressing, tape, wrap, or net ▪ Aren't recommended for nondraining wounds ▪ May cause maceration of skin surrounding wound if not changed regularly

Dressing type	Indications for use	Advantages	Disadvantages
Hydrocolloids (Used as a primary or secondary dressing)	▪ Partial- to full-thickness wounds ▪ Wounds with minimal to moderate drainage ▪ Wounds with necrosis or slough	▪ Nonadherent to a moist wound base ▪ Conform easily to the wound bed ▪ Maintain moisture by becoming gelatinous as they absorb drainage ▪ May be left in place up to 7 days, depending on wound characteristics ▪ Can easily be removed from the wound base ▪ Come in several forms and in both thin and traditional thicknesses ▪ Promote autolytic debridement ▪ Impermeable to water and bacteria	▪ May have an odor when removed ▪ Can't be used on burns or dry wounds ▪ Can cause skin stripping when removed ▪ Can cause maceration or hypergranulation ▪ May need to be held in place to maximize adhesion ▪ Aren't recommended for wounds with heavy drainage, sinus tracts, tunneling, or fragile periwound skin
Hydrogels (Gel or impregnated gauze forms are used as primary dressings; sheets are used as primary or secondary dressings)	▪ Partial- to full-thickness wounds ▪ Dry wounds ▪ Wounds with minimal drainage ▪ Wounds with necrosis or slough ▪ Infected wounds	▪ Available in sheet, strip, impregnated gauze, and amorphous gel forms ▪ Cool wounds to ease pain ▪ Add moisture to wounds ▪ Promote autolytic debridement ▪ Are easy to apply and remove ▪ Can be used to fill cavities or tunnels (gel or impregnated gauze forms)	▪ Require a secondary dressing (gel and impregnated gauze forms) ▪ Can macerate surrounding skin ▪ May necessitate daily dressing changes ▪ Not recommended for wounds with heavy drainage

(continued)

Wound care dressing review (continued)

Dressing type	Indications for use	Advantages	Disadvantages
Specialty absorptives (Used as a primary or secondary dressing)	▪ Infected or noninfected wounds with heavy drainage	▪ Are highly absorbent ▪ Typically require less frequent changes ▪ Are available in various forms ▪ Are easy to apply and remove	▪ Can't be used on burns or on wounds with little or no drainage
Transparent films (Used as a primary or secondary dressing)	▪ Partial-thickness wounds with minimal exudate ▪ Wounds with eschar (to promote autolysis)	▪ May require less-frequent changes ▪ Allow visualization of the wound ▪ Aren't bulky ▪ Are impermeable to bacteria	▪ Don't absorb drainage ▪ Can strip the skin when removed; not for use on fragile skin ▪ Can be difficult to handle and apply
Wound fillers (Used as a primary dressing)	▪ Infected and noninfected wounds ▪ Wounds with minimal to moderate drainage ▪ Wounds requiring packing	▪ Available in several forms with different capabilities ▪ Can fill dead space in wounds ▪ Are easy to apply and remove	▪ Require a secondary dressing ▪ Can't be used on third-degree burns or dry wounds ▪ Can alarm some patients because of the wormlike appearance of some products

Other treatments

Topical drugs and other treatments can complement the function of dressings to promote wound healing.

> Cross-hatching helps to ensure that the debriding agent penetrates the tissue so that it can begin to liquefy and digest necrotic tissue.

Debriding agents

Chemical or enzyme preparations called *debriding agents* are topically applied to necrotic or devitalized tissue to help facilitate its removal from a wound.

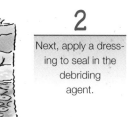

Necrotic tissue

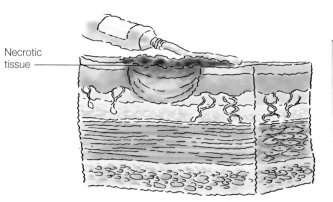

1

First, apply the debriding agent to the surface of the wound after cross-hatching any eschar (scoring it with a scalpel in a meshlike pattern).

2

Next, apply a dressing to seal in the debriding agent.

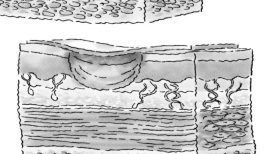

3

Once or twice daily, remove the dressing and irrigate the wound to remove the liquefied necrotic material. Afterward, apply more debriding agent and a clean dressing.

Negative pressure wound therapy

When a wound fails to heal in a timely manner, negative pressure wound therapy may be used. Vacuum-assisted closure (VAC), an example of this type of therapy system, requires a special dressing, a vacuum tube, and a vacuum pump.

Vacuum-assisted closure

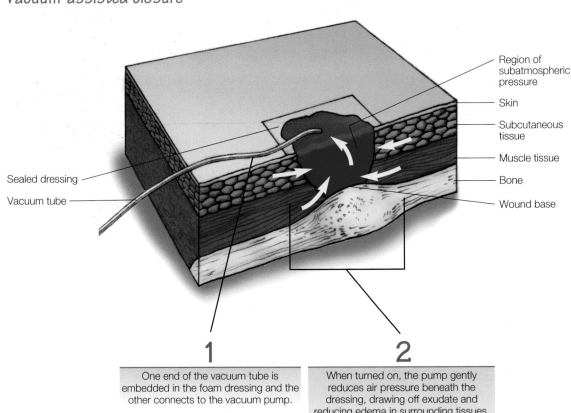

1
One end of the vacuum tube is embedded in the foam dressing and the other connects to the vacuum pump.

2
When turned on, the pump gently reduces air pressure beneath the dressing, drawing off exudate and reducing edema in surrounding tissues. This process reduces bacterial colonization, promotes granulation tissue development, increases the rate of cell mitosis, and spurs the migration of epithelial cells within the wound.

Choosing a VAC dressing

The dressing used with a vacuum-assisted closure (VAC) device varies, depending upon the wound being treated.

> Choosing which dressing to use with VAC isn't always a black or white issue. For example, either dressing may be suitable for treating diabetic ulcers, dry wounds, skin grafts, shallow chronic wounds, and deep trauma wounds.

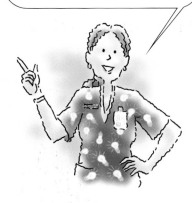

Black foam dressing

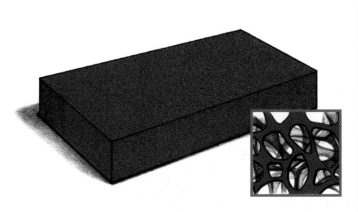

Benefits

The open, porous structure of this polyurethane dressing:
- stimulates the formation of granulation tissue
- evenly distributes negative pressure throughout the wound
- facilitates the removal of drainage.

Indications
- Deep acute wounds
- Deep pressure ulcers
- Flaps

White foam dressing

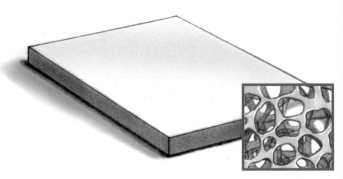

Benefits

This dense dressing made of a microporous polyvinyl alcohol material:
- reduces the growth of granulation tissue into the dressing (which reduces the pain of dressing changes)
- protects delicate structures
- prevents wound adherence.

Indications
- Wounds with sufficient granulation tissue
- Wounds with tunnels, sinus tracts, or areas of undermining
- Superficial wounds
- Painful wounds

Applying a VAC dressing

3

Apply the pad with tubing over the hole made in the drape.

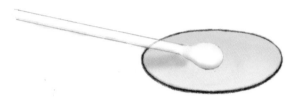

2

Cut the drape to extend 1¹/₄" to 2" (3 to 5 cm) over adjacent skin in all directions. Make a small hole in the center. Seal the drape securely.

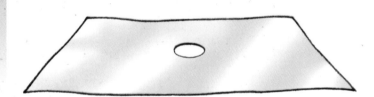

1

Cut the foam dressing to fit the size and shape of the wound, extending it into areas of tunneling or undermining.

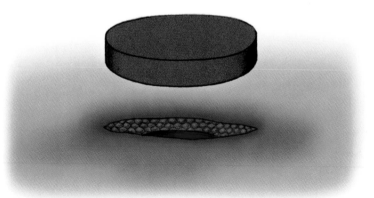

Provant wound-closure system

The Provant wound-closure system emits a radiofrequency signal into a wound to induce production of fibroblasts and epithelial cells and to trigger the secretion of multiple growth factors. This promotes wound healing, even in cases of chronic, severe pressure ulcers.

1

A treatment application pad (protected by a disposable cover) is placed over the wound. The dressing doesn't have to be removed.

2

The pad directs a radio-frequency signal $2^3/4''$ to $3^1/4''$ (7 to 8 cm) into the tissues around the wound. The signal triggers the:

- proliferation of fibroblasts, necessary for the development of granulation tissue
- proliferation of epithelial cells, necessary for wound closure
- secretion of multiple growth factors, to speed healing
- expression and activation of hundreds of genes controlling inflammation, granulation, epithelialization, and remodeling.

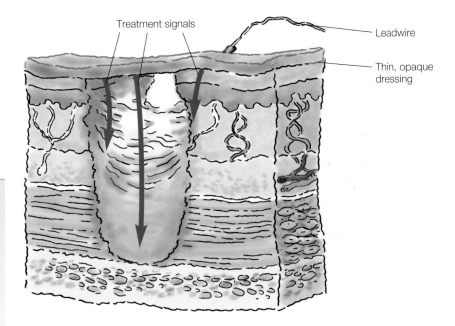

Treatment signals

Leadwire

Thin, opaque dressing

Growth factor therapy

Growth factor therapy is a type of biotherapy used to stimulate cell proliferation in wound treatment. The growth factor must be synthesized, secreted, and removed from the tissues at the correct time to prevent stalling of wound healing. It should be applied using a sterile applicator, such as a swab or tongue blade, or saline-moistened gauze. Then the wound should be dressed with saline-moistened gauze.

Honey therapy

In honey therapy, a dressing composed of glucose oxidase and active *Leptospermum* honey (a medical-grade honey) is applied to the skin. Honey has antibacterial properties due to its high sugar content, low moisture content, gluconic acid, and peroxide.

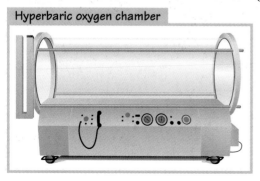

And I thought honey was only good on toast!

Hyperbaric oxygen therapy

Hyperbaric oxygen therapy involves the delivery of 100% oxygen through a sealed chamber. A total body chamber increases the amount of dissolved oxygen in the blood that's available for wound healing.

Hyperbaric oxygen chamber

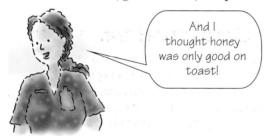

Understanding growth factors

Type	Description
TGF-β (transforming growth factor beta)	Controls movement of cells to sites of inflammation and stimulates extracellular matrix formation
bFGF (basic fibroblast growth factor)	Stimulates angiogenesis (the development of blood vessels)
VEGF (vascular endothelial growth factor)	Stimulates angiogenesis
IGF (insulin-like growth factor)	Increases collagen synthesis
EGF (epidermal growth factor)	Stimulates epidermal regeneration

Pulsatile lavage

Pulsatile lavage is a form of hydrotherapy that can be used with almost any wound type. It involves the application of room temperature sterile normal saline solution to the wound bed under pressure using a spray gun with simultaneous aspiration of the solution by negative pressure through a separate tube in the gun.

Pulsatile lavage gun

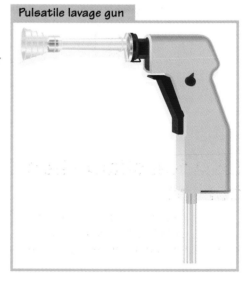

Ultraviolet radiation therapy

Ultraviolet (UV) radiation therapy is used to treat slowly healing wounds, necrotic wounds, and infected or heavily contaminated wounds.

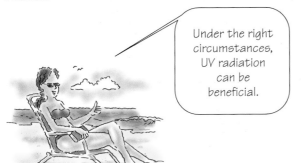

Under the right circumstances, UV radiation can be beneficial.

UVC radiation device

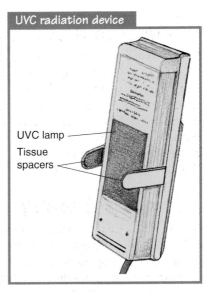

UVC lamp

Tissue spacers

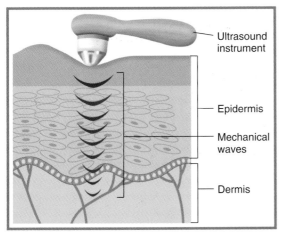

Ultrasound instrument

Epidermis

Mechanical waves

Dermis

Ultrasound treatment

In ultrasound treatment, mechanical pressure waves are used to hasten healing and help decrease pain and inflammation. Optimal effects are seen when this treatment is used during the inflammatory phase of wound healing.

Electrical stimulation device

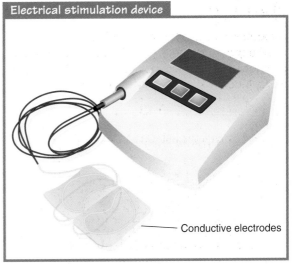

Conductive electrodes

Electrical stimulation treatment

In electrical stimulation, electrical current is delivered by conductive electrodes to the skin or to the skin and a wound to enhance healing.

Review of other wound care treatments

Use this chart to quickly review the indications for use, advantages, and disadvantages of other wound care treatments.

Drug or device	Indications for use	Advantages	Disadvantages
Debriding agents	• Wounds with moderate to large amounts of necrotic tissue • Wounds in which surgical debridement is contraindicated	• May contain chlorophyll, which helps control odor • Debride effectively even when used in small amounts	• May contain known allergens • May require secondary dressings • May irritate surrounding skin • May cause a burning sensation in the wound that can last for several hours • May turn drainage green (if product contains chlorophyll), leading to false concern of infection
Negative pressure wound theraphy	• Slow-healing acute, subacute, or chronic exudative wounds with cavities • Pressure ulcers or surgical wounds more than 1 cm deep	• Cleans deeply and can manage moderate to large amounts of drainage • Can manage multiple wounds when dressings are cut to bridge two or more wounds • May allow patient mobility (some models have rechargeable batteries and are small enough to fit in a pouch worn at the waist or over the shoulder)	• Is contraindicated for untreated osteomyelitis, malignancies, and wounds with necrotic tissue or fistulas • Impairs mobility (vacuum tube is 5′ to 6′ [1.5 to 2 m] long) • Requires electricity or rechargeable batteries to operate • Can cause bruising at the wound base if the pressure is improperly set
Provant wound-closure system	• Wounds in the inflammatory phase of healing	• Requires no special training (patients can perform therapy at home) • Requires only two 30-minute treatments per day (device turns off automatically at the end of a session) • May be used over existing dressings	• Is contraindicated for use in pregnant patients and patients with cardiac pacemakers • Won't promote healing of bone or deep internal organs
Becaplermin growth factor therapy – Example: Platelet-derived growth factor becaplermin (Regranex)	• Full-thickness diabetic neuropathic ulcers that have adequate blood flow • Clean, noninfected, granulating wounds	• Provides growth factors needed for wound healing • Attracts fibroblasts and induces them to divide, which aids wound healing • Must be applied only once daily • Requires no special training for application	• Can't be used on necrotic tissue or infected wounds • Is contraindicated in patients with poor blood supply to the legs or neoplasms near the wound • May cause a localized rash
Honey therapy	• Burns • Ophthalmic conditions • GI tract problems • Periodontal disease • Surgical wounds • Wound barrier against tumor implantation in laparoscopic gynecological surgery	• Improves wound healing time • Reduces scar formation	• May result in an allergy to bee proteins or pollen (rare)

Review of other wound care treatments *(continued)*

Drug or device	Indications for use	Advantages	Disadvantages
Hyperbaric oxygen therapy	▪ Diabetic foot ulcers and poorly healing venous ulcers that haven't improved with traditional therapies	▪ Enhances the activity of neutrophils ▪ Relieves relative hypoxia in wound tissues	▪ Is contraindicated in patients taking antineoplastic agents and those with known pneumothorax
Pulsatile lavage	▪ Infected or heavily contaminated wounds ▪ Wounds that require preparation for grafting with either skin grafts or living skin equivalents ▪ Wounds that require removal of necrotic tissue or other particulate matter	▪ Increases granulation tissue formation in clean and slow-healing wounds ▪ Decreases bioburden levels in infected or heavily contaminated wounds ▪ Is less uncomfortable than some other treatments ▪ Is easily accessible due to portability of the equipment ▪ Is effective in reaching deep, tunneling wounds ▪ Minimizes cross-contamination	▪ Requires the use of low impact and suction pressure on fragile tissue and avoiding direct pressure over exposed nerves and blood vessels
Ultraviolet radiation therapy	▪ Chronic, slow healing wounds ▪ Infected or heavily contaminated wounds ▪ Necrotic wounds	*UVA and UVB radiation* ▪ Increases wound healing in chronic pressure ulcers ▪ Enhances white blood cell (WBC) accumulation and lysosomal activity in wounds ▪ Increases production of interleukin-1 alpha (a cytokine involved in epithelialization) *UVC radiation* ▪ Kills a broad spectrum of microorganisms with low exposure times ▪ Is quickly and easily administered	▪ Is contraindicated in patients with a history of skin cancer, diabetes, pulmonary tuberculosis, hyperthyroidism, systemic lupus erythematosus, acute eczema, herpes simplex, or cardiac, renal, or hepatic disease
Ultrasound treatment	▪ Open and closed wounds	▪ Is portable ▪ Requires only a short application time ▪ Doesn't require dependent positioning ▪ Involves no risk of maceration ▪ Reduces bioburden ▪ Increases WBC migration to the wound bed ▪ Promotes orderly arrangement of collagen in wounds	▪ May require several treatment sessions (for large wounds) ▪ May be painful or difficult to apply over irregular surfaces ▪ Increases the risk of wound contamination
Electrical stimulation	▪ Recalcitrant wounds, especially chronic pressure ulcers	▪ Promotes cellular migration ▪ Enhances blood flow ▪ Increases protein synthesis and wound bed formation ▪ Destroys microorganisms ▪ Increases angiogenesis and tissue oxygenation ▪ Reduces wound bioburden, microbial content, and wound and diabetic neuropathic pain	▪ Can't be used on malignant tissue ▪ Can't be used over the pericardial area, other areas related to control of cardiac and respiratory function, or implanted devices ▪ Is contraindicated in patients with untreated osteomyelitis

VISION QUEST

My word!

Use the clues to help you unscramble the names of three types of wound dressings. Then use the circled letters to answer the question posed.

Question: Controlling the amount of moisture in a wound is crucial for what to occur?

1. These dressings contain multiple layers of highly absorbent material, such as cotton or rayon.

spaceylit vaporsbite

— —◯— — — —◯— —   ◯— — — — — — — — —

2. Made from seaweed, these dressings contain very soft, nonwoven fibers that turn into a biodegradable gel as they absorb exudate.

alientag — —◯—◯— — —

3. These adhesive, moldable wafers are impermeable to oxygen, water, and water vapor.

coldhydrooil ◯— — — — — — — — —◯—

Answer: — — — — — — —

Show and tell

Describe the steps for applying a debiriding agent to a wound based on the images shown.

1. _____
_____
_____
_____

2. _____
_____
_____
_____

3. _____
_____
_____
_____

194

Answers: My word! 1. Specially absorptive, 2. Alginate, 3. Hydrocolloid; Question: Healing; Show and tell 1. Apply the debriding agent to the wound's surface. 2. Apply a dressing to seal in the debriding agent. 3. Remove the dressing and irrigate the wound once or twice daily.

Selected references

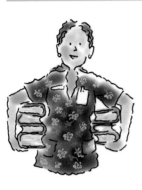

Andersen, A. S., et al. (2010). A novel approach to the antimicrobial activity of maggot debridement therapy. *Journal of Antimicrobial Chemotherapy, 65*(8), 1646–1654.

Baranoski, S., & Ayello, E. A. (2008). *Wound care essentials: Practice principles* (2nd ed.). Philadelphia, PA: Lippincott Williams & Wilkins.

Bell, C., & McCarthy, G. (2010). The assessment and treatment of wound pain at dressing change. *British Journal of Nursing, 19*(11), S4, S6, S8 passim.

Brown, P. (2009). *Quick reference to wound care* (3rd ed.). Sudbury, MA: Jones and Bartlett Pubs.

Bryant, R. A., & Nix, D. P. (2011). *Acute and chronic wounds: Current management concepts* (4th ed.). St. Louis, MO: Mosby Elsevier.

Chang, J., & Cuellar, N. G. (2009). The use of honey for wound care management: A traditional remedy revisited. *Home Healthcare Nurse, 27*(5), 308–316.

Choi, M., Armstrong, M. B., & Panthaki, Z. J. (2009). Pediatric hand burns: Thermal, electrical, chemical. *Journal of Craniofacial Surgery, 20*(4), 1045–1048.

Fauci, A. S., et al. (2008). *Harrison's principles of internal medicine* (17th ed.). New York, NY: McGraw-Hill Co.

Hall, B. J., & Hall, J. C. (Eds.). (2010). *Sauer's manual of skin diseases* (10th ed.). Philadelphia, PA: Lippincott Williams & Wilkins.

Kirsner, R. S. (2010). Biological agents for chronic wounds. *American Journal of Clinical Dermatology, 11* (Suppl. 1), 23–25.

Langemo, D. K., et al. (2009). Use of honey for wound healing. *Advances in Skin & Wound Care, 22*(3), 113–118.

Löndahl, M., et al. (2010). Hyperbaric oxygen therapy facilitates healing of chronic foot ulcers in patients with diabetes. *Diabetes Care, 33*(5), 998–1003.

Moore, K., et al. (2010). Surface bacteriology of venous leg ulcers and healing outcome. *Journal of Clinical Pathology, 63*(9), 830–834.

Pandey, M., Kumar, P., & Khanna, A. K. (2009). Marjolin's ulcer associated with chronic osteomyelitis. *Journal of Wound Care, 18*(12), 504–506.

Pieper, B. (2009). Honey-based dressings and wound care: An option for care in the United States. *Journal of Wound, Ostomy, and Continence Nursing, 36*(1), 60–66.

Shaikh, N., et al. (2010). Hospital epidemiology of emergent cervical necrotizing fasciitis. *Journal of Emergencies, Trauma & Shock, 3*(2), 123–125.

Smith, T., Legel, K., & Hanft, J. R. (2009). Topical *Leptospermum* honey (Medihoney) in recalcitrant venous leg wounds: A preliminary case series. *Advances in Skin & Wound Care, 22*(2), 68–71.

Snyder, S. M., Beshlian, K. M., & Hampson, N. B. (2010). Hyperbaric oxygen and reduction mammaplasty in the previously irradiated breast. *Plastic and Reconstructive Surgery, 125*(6), 255e–257e.

Tavernelli, K., Reif, S., & Larsen, T. (2010). Managing venous leg ulcers in the home. *Ostomy Wound Management, 56*(2), 10–12.

Yantis, M. A., O'Toole, K. N., & Ring, P. (2009). Leech therapy. *American Journal of Nursing, 109*(4), 36–42.

Credits

Chapter 1
Epidermal layers, page 4. Premkumar, K. (2004). *The massage connection anatomy and physiology.* Baltimore, MD: Lippincott Williams & Wilkins.

Blood supply, page 5. Rubin, E., & Farber, J. L. (1999). *Pathology* (3rd ed.). Philadelphia, PA: Lippincott Williams & Wilkins.

Chapter 3
Stage III pressure ulcer, page 37. Reprinted with permission from the National Pressure Ulcer Advisory Panel slide series #1. Available: *www.npuap.org.*

Chapter 4
Cleaning a wound, pages 40-41; Packing a wound, page 45; Hydrocolloid dressing, page 48; Moist saline gauze, page 49. Lynn, P. (2007). *Taylor's clinical nursing skills: A nursing process approach.* Philadelphia, PA: Lippincott Williams & Wilkins.

Nonviable tissue and healthy tissue, page 54. Maggot larva, page 55. Fleisher, G. R., et al. (2004). *Atlas of pediatric emergency medicine.* Philadelphia, PA: Lippincott Williams & Wilkins.

Chapter 5
Sunburn, page 60; Superficial partial-thickness burn, page 62; Postoperative leg infection, page 73. Images provided by Stedman's.

Partial-thickness sunburn, page 62; Deep partial-thickness burns, page 63; Full-thickness burn, page 65 (top). Fleisher, G. R., et al. (2004). *Atlas of pediatric emergency medicine.* Philadelphia, PA: Lippincott Williams & Wilkins.

Third-degree hand and wrist burn, page 65 (middle); Third-degree foot burn, page 65 (bottom). © English, MD/Custom Medical Stock Photo.

Electrical burn, page 66 (bottom). Rubin, E., & Farber, J. L. (1999). *Pathology* (3rd ed.). Philadelphia, PA: Lippincott Williams & Wilkins.

Types of skin grafts, page 70, and Common donor sites, page 71. Smeltzer, S. C., & Bare, B. G. (2003). *Brunner and Suddarth's textbook of medical-surgical nursing* (10th ed.). Philadelphia, PA: Lippincott Williams & Wilkins.

Dermatome, page 71. © English, MD/Custom Medical Stock Photo.

Chapter 6
Braden scale, pages 90 and 91. Copyright 1988. Barbara Braden and Nancy Bergstrom. Reprinted with permission. All rights reserved. Permission to use this tool in clinical practice may be obtained, usually free of charge, at *www.bradenscale.com.*

Norton scale, page 92. Doreen Norton, Rhoda McLaren, & A.N. Exton-Smith, *An Investigation of Geriatric Nursing Problems in Hospital.* Copyright National Corporation for the Care of Old People (now Centre for Policy on Ageing), London, 1962.

Support surface characteristics, page 95; Suspected deep tissue injury, p. 99; Management of pressure ulcers algorithm, page 103; Nutritional assessment and support algorithm, page 104; Management of tissue loads algorithm, page 105; Managing bacterial colonization and infection algorithm, page 106. Agency for Healthcare Policy and Research, National Library of Medicine. (1994). Treatment of Pressure Ulcers: Clinical Practice Guideline Number 15 (AHCPR Publication Number 95-0652). Retrieved from http://www.ncbi.nlm.nih.gov/bookshelf/br.fcgi?book=hsahcpr&part=A5124.

PUSH tool, page 98. Copyright National Pressure Ulcer Advisory Panel, 1998. Adapted with permission.

Deep tissue injury, page 99. Courtesy of Joyce M. Black, PhD, RN. Associate Professor, University of Nebraska Medical Center, College of Nursing.

Pressure ulcers, stages I to IV, pages 100–102. Nettina, S. M. (2001). *The Lippincott manual of nursing practice* (7th ed.). Philadelphia, PA: Lippincott Williams & Wilkins.

Chapter 7
Lymphatic system, page 116. Premkumar, K. (2004). *The massage connection: Anatomy and physiology.* Baltimore, MD: Lippincott Williams & Wilkins.

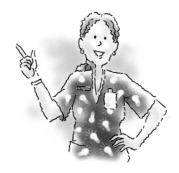

Venous stasis ulcer, page 121 (left); Stasis dermatitis with venous ulcer, page 122 (top). Goodheart, H. P. (2003). *Goodheart's photoguide of common skin disorders* (2nd ed.). Philadelphia, PA: Lippincott Williams & Wilkins.

Chronic venous ulcer, page 121 (right); Advanced chronic venous ulcer, page 122 (bottom); Arterial insufficiency, page 126 (left). Marks, R. (1987). *Skin disease in old age.* Philadelphia, PA: J.B. Lippincott.

Venous stasis ulcer, page 122 (middle). Weber, J., & Kelley, J. (2003). *Health assessment in nursing* (2nd ed.). Philadelphia, PA: Lippincott Williams & Wilkins.

Arterial emboli ulcers, page 125; Gangrene, page 126 (right). Smeltzer, S. C., & Bare, B. G. (2003). *Brunner and Suddarth's textbook of medical-surgical nursing* (10th ed.). Philadelphia, PA: Lippincott Williams & Wilkins.

Lymphedema, page 127. Rubin, E., & Farber, J. L. (1999). *Pathology* (3rd ed.). Philadelphia, PA: Lippincott Williams & Wilkins.

Signs of lymphedema, page 128. Bickley L. S., & Szilagyi, P. (2003). *Bates' guide to physical examination and history taking* (8th ed.). Philadelphia, PA: Lippincott Williams & Wilkins.

Treatment of arterial ulcers algorithm, page 132. Adapted with permission from Arterial vs. venous ulcers: Diagnosis and treatment (2001, May-June). *Advances in Skin & Wound Care, 14*(3), 147.

Chapter 8

Neuropathic ulcer, page 142 (left). Marks, R. (1987). *Skin disease in old age.* Philadelphia, PA: J. B. Lippincott.

Diabetic heel ulcer, page 142 (right). Goodheart, H. P. (2003). *Goodheart's photoguide of common skin disorders* (2nd ed.). Philadelphia, PA: Lippincott Williams & Wilkins.

University of Texas Diabetic Foot Classification System, page 143. Adapted with permission from Armstrong, D. G., et al. (1996). Treatment-based classification system for assessment and care of diabetic feet. *JAPMA, 86*(7), 311–316.

Wagner Ulcer Grade Classification, page 143. Adapted with permission from Wagner, F. W., Jr. (1987). The diabetic foot. *Orthopedics, 10,* 163–172. © SLACK Incorporated.

Treatment algorithm for diabetic ulcers, page 144; Wound care algorithm for diabetic ulcers, page 145. Adapted with permission from *Advances in Skin & Wound Care, 13*(1), 35, January-February 2000.

Chapter 9

Squamous cell carcinoma, pages 151 and 153. Goodheart, H. P. (2003). *Goodheart's photoguide of common skin disorders* (2nd ed.). Philadelphia, PA: Lippincott Williams & Wilkins.

Basal cell carcinoma, page 151. Rubin, E., & Farber, J. L. (1999). *Pathology* (3rd ed.). Philadelphia, PA: Lippincott Williams & Wilkins.

Inflamed carcinoma of breast, page 152. Moore, K. L., & Agur, A. (2002). *Essential clinical anatomy* (2nd ed.). Philadelphia, PA: Lippincott Williams & Wilkins.

Metastatic lymphoma, page 152. Image provided by Stedman's.

Chapter 10

Spider bite, page 158. Courtesy of George A. Datto III, MD.

Dog bite, page 158. From Fleisher, G. R., Ludwig, W., & Baskin, M. N. (2004). *Atlas of pediatric emergency medicine.* Philadelphia, PA: Lippincott Williams & Wilkins.

Intravenous extravasation ulcer, page 159. From Strickland, J. W., & Graham, T. J. (2005). *Master techniques in orthopedic surgery: The hand* (2nd ed.). Philadelphia, PA: Lippincott Williams & Wilkins.

Necrotizing fasciitis, page 160. Image provided by Stedman's.

Pyoderma gangrenosum ulcer, page 160; Systemic lupus erythematosus ulcer, page 161. Goodheart, H. P. (2003). *Goodheart's photoguide of common skin disorders* (2nd ed.). Philadelphia, PA: Lippincott Williams & Wilkins.

Scleroderma, page 161. Image provided by Stedman's.

Thromboangiitis obliterans, page 162. Rubin, E., & Farber, J. L. (1999). *Pathology* (3rd ed.). Philadelphia, PA: Lippincott Williams & Wilkins.

Warfarin-induced necrosis, page 162. Reprinted with permission from eMedicine.com, 2010. Available at: *http://em=dicine.medscape.com/article/1096183-overview*

We gratefully acknowledge Anatomical Chart Company and LifeART for the use of selected images.

Index

A

Abdominal binder for bariatric patients, 79
Absorbable sutures, 76
Absorption as skin function, 6
Acetic acid, 43
Acute wound, characteristics of, 24
Adhesive wound closures, 75
Advanced age, pressure ulcer risk and, 89
Aging
  effects of, on wound healing, 17
  skin function and, 7
Air-fluidized therapy bed, 95
Alginate dressing, 133
  advantages of, 181
  application method for, 48
  disadvantages of, 181
  indications for, 181
  removal of, 168
Algorithm
  for arterial ulcer treatment, 132
  for bacterial colonization and infection management in pressure ulcers, 106
  for diabetic ulcer treatment, 144
  for diabetic ulcer wound care, 145
  for dressing a wound, 47
  for nutritional assessment and support for pressure ulcer patient, 104
  for pressure ulcer management, 103
  for pressure ulcer prevention, 94
  for reassessment, 42
  for tissue load management of pressure ulcers, 105
  for venous ulcer treatment, 130
Allograft, 70
Alternating pressure mattress, 95, 96
Amniotic membrane dressing, 69
Anaerobic specimen, collecting, 52
Ankle-brachial index (ABI), 118
Antimicrobial dressings, 169
  advantages of, 181
  disadvantages of, 181
  indications for, 181
  mechanics of, 170
Antiseptic solutions for wound cleaning, 43
Arterial insufficiency
  causes of, 123
  risk factors for, 123
  signs of, 124

Arterial ulcers, 119, 123–126
  algorithm for, 132
  arterial insufficiency and, 124
  atherosclerosis and, 123
  characteristics of, 126–127
  clinical findings in, 119
  development of, 123
  dressings for, 133
  therapies and procedures for, 129
  treatment goals for, 129
  treatment of, 129
  typical locations of, 119
  wound care for, 129
Arteries, 112–114
  assessing blood flow through, 114
  in lower limb, 113
Atherosclerosis, arterial ulcers and, 123
Atypical wounds
  causes, 158
  treatments, 163
  types, 158–162
Autograft, 70
Autolytic debridement, 53

B

Bacterial colonization and infection management for pressure ulcers, algorithm for, 106
Bariatric patients, wound care in, 79
Becaplermin growth factor therapy, wound care, 190, 192
Biobrane dressing, 69
Biologic debridement, 53, 55–56
Biological dressings, 69
  advantages of, 181
  disadvantages of, 181
  indications for, 181
Bites, atypical wounds, 158
Black widow spider bite, 163
Black wounds, 29, 30
Blanket continuous suture, 76
Blebs, evacuating, from sheet graft, 72
Blood supply for skin, 5
Body surface area, burn estimation and, 67, 68
Braden scale for pressure ulcer risk assessment, 90–91
Brown recluse spider bite, 163
Burns, 60–73
  biological dressings for, 69
  electrical, 66
  estimating extent of, 67–68

Burns *(continued)*
  first-degree, 60
  full-thickness, 64–65
  second-degree, 61–63
  deep partial-thickness, 61, 63
  superficial partial-thickness, 61, 62
  skin grafts for, 70–73
  third-degree, 64–65
Butterfly wound closures, 75

C

Cadaver dressings, 69
Cancer patient, malignant wounds in, 150
Capillaries
  blood supply to skin and, 5
  lymphedema and, 127
Charcot's disease, sensory neuropathy and, 137, 142
Chemical debridement, 53
Chlorhexidine, 43
Chronic wound, characteristics of, 24
Circular wound, cleaning technique for, 41
Cleaning a wound, 40–43
  antiseptic solutions for, 43
  choosing agent for, 43
  reassessment after, 42
  techniques for, 41
Closed-wound drainage system, 80
Collagen dressings, 171
  advantages of, 181
  disadvantages of, 181
  indications for, 181
Color of wound, 27–30
  tailoring care to, 30
Colostomy care, 81–83
Compartment syndrome, 73
Composite dressings, 172
  advantages of, 182
  disadvantages of, 182
  indications for, 182
Compression system, inelastic, 131
Contact layer dressings, 173
  advantages of, 182
  disadvantages of, 182
  indications for, 182

D

Dakin's solution, 43
Debriding a wound, 53–56
  methods for, 53
Debriding agents, 185, 192